LOOKING GOOD

LOOKING GOOD

A GUIDE FOR MEN

CHARLES HIX

Photographs by Bruce Weber

Drawings by Kas Sable

HAWTHORN BOOKS, INC.
Publishers / New York

LOOKING GOOD

Library of Congress Catalog Card Number: 76–41975

ISBN: 0–8015–4670–2

1 2 3 4 5 6 7 8 9 10

To   *George Mazzei,*
        who more than any other editor helped me get this far;

        David Platt,
        who suggested to Hawthorn Books that I write this book;

        Sandra Choron,
        who took his recommendation, thank heavens (and Sandra, too);

        Bruce Weber,
        who came through when my heart was sinking;

        Brian Burdine,
        who, hung over on a Monday, still had perfect vision;

        and *R.D.,*
        who is always there.

CONTENTS

FACE

THE BODY

HANDS & FEET

ACKNOWLEDGMENTS

Many must be thanked, but my acknowledgments must be a bit unconventional. During the years I've spent writing about men's grooming, many people have helped both directly and indirectly, and if I hadn't known them, I could not have written *Looking Good.*

First, I'd like to thank the staff of *Gentlemen's Quarterly,* especially its former managing editor, George Mazzei. Some of the material in this book first appeared in altered (and occasionally not-so-altered) form in that magazine. Jack Haber, *GQ*s editor, arranged for me to use the material. Thank you.

While I was a novice in the grooming field, certain individuals made special contributions. Although I may not have been in contact with some of them recently, I feel their presence in what I've written. I'm especially grateful to Mario Badescu, who introduced me to the intricacies of skin care; Amelia Bassin, who proved to me that men's fragrance can be both fascinating and fun; Kenneth Battelle, probably the world's most famous and exclusive hairdresser, who took the time to teach me about hair; Susan Biehn and

Andy Lucarelli, simply for being particularly encouraging and honest; Dr. Joyce Brothers, for offering me insights into why men were (and too often still are) skittish about grooming; and Pennye Pennix, who led the way to my understanding of skin care for blacks.

Three dermatologists, Dr. Robert Berger, Dr. Ronald Sherman, and Dr. Diane Tanenbaum, and one plastic surgeon, Dr. James Stallings, although not interviewed specifically for this book, nonetheless have given me invaluable assistance during previous conversations.

While most companies were helpful (let's hear a raspberry for those who weren't), some went extra miles. In particular, I bow to Barbara Gleason at Aramis, Sy Sperling at Hair Club for Men, Ron Barris and John Zervoulei at Headstart Hair for Men, Geri Brin at Norelco, and Beverly Hines at Scannon. And I must thank that wiz of a hair stylist, Marilyn Sheinberg. Thanks, too, to Maureen Logan at Dorothy Gray.

On a personal note, four special people lived through this experience with me, Susan Leslie, Victoria Meekins, Susan (the Songbird from Chicago)

O'Neill, and Bob Dahlin. Thank you all for being part of my life and for helping me muddle through.

Of course, I truly want to acknowledge the keen contributions of my editor, Sandra Choron, who may not possess the patience of a saint but who is an angel nevertheless.

Lastly, I am deeply grateful to the models who were generous with their time, and especially to Phil at Lexington Labs, the photo studio that did such a fine job of printing the photographs for the book: After putting so much of himself behind the camera, Bruce deserved the best and got it.

INTRODUCTION

My father isn't a prince—or even a count. My mother hasn't hoarded family beauty secrets that have been passed from generation to generation. I was raised to believe that soap and water are next to godliness, but otherwise not to worry.

So how does it happen that I've written a book about men's grooming? I cringe at even the thought of belabored life stories, so I'll try to keep this brief.

About eight years ago I became fed up with working for a giant textiles company. Since I wasn't thirty yet, I figured I could just quit and see what happened. Not necessarily a very practical decision, but I risked it. I'd worked on a newspaper before that, so I thought I'd try free-lance writing. The first magazine assignment I received was to write a long piece about the "peacock revolution" (how dated that phrase seems now) in men's grooming. I had fun with it, wrote an amusing piece, sharpening some barbs. That's how men's grooming was treated in those days and often still is. The piece received some attention. Overnight I became a grooming "expert." I started doing more articles on men's grooming and fashion.

Then it dawned on me that maybe I'd better learn something about my new-found field.

After interviewing literally hundreds of other "experts" about the "right" approach to grooming, I found that my mind was boggled. No two experts agreed. Pretty soon I realized that whereas some experts were innocently misinformed, others were deliberately trying to misinform me in order to promote their own products or services.

I also learned that a lot still isn't known about personal care and that the ongoing battle between physicians, aestheticians, and the cosmetics industry often clouds, not clarifies, the issues. A believer in plain old common sense, I set about sifting through various claims and counterclaims in order to examine them in the light of logic. I hope I've been successful. I can't sign a contract in blood swearing that my conclusions will work for every man. I'm not a doctor, a cosmetician, or a scientist; I'm a writer. But I can guarantee that I haven't been swayed by any vested interest. To be fair, I've tried to present opposing viewpoints on controversial grooming issues.

I've been using that word *grooming* a lot. I don't like it; it's something you do to a horse. But I haven't found a better word. If you have one, let me know.

One of the toughest aspects about this book was naming it. Although it's expected that women will try even the weirdest concoctions to improve their looks (sorry if that sounds sexist), that a man should do anything at all in the same interest has often been suspect. Ah, the double standards! From infancy a male is trained *not* to look in a mirror except as a hasty once-over before rushing out the front door. A sign of vanity, you know. Yet, isn't it a peculiarly perverse type of vanity when a guy will purposefully disregard self-care so others will consider him "masculine"? Is unhealthy skin masculine? After all, good grooming, while it makes you look better, is based on maintaining every part of the body at its healthiest. True, grooming also includes decisions about how best to style your hair or whether or not to grow a beard. But the first priority for looking good remains straightforward cleanliness, not elaborate camouflage.

Obviously, if clean living is the prerequisite of good health and good grooming, overindulgence of any kind is bad. Drugs, alcohol, and tobacco don't do anything good for the body, so their use is discouraged. Our organisms are nourished by the food we eat, so bad eating habits won't feed a good appearance. Unexercised bodies become flabby. But we all know these things. Why preach? Do what you will, I'm not a parole officer. Hell, I smoke and have been known to tipple a martini or two. I realize, in the long run , I could look better and feel better if I didn't; but in the short term, I have no pretensions about sainthood. I do wish I could improve my tennis game.

I also wish I possessed some universal key to inner happiness for mankind. Womankind, too. Emotional stress and distress work as hard against looking good as bad habits and benign neglect. Internal turmoil leaves its mark on the exterior. Loving helps; hating hurts. The world would be both prettier and handsomer if we could all get ourselves together. Who cares how it's accomplished if only it is? The routes will be different for different men. Find your own and travel it happily.

There's no formula for looking good. The work is steady but not arduous. The most rigorous part may be training yourself to think logically about what you're doing and why. One of the worst sins that beauty magazines commit is their commandments to use this cream or that lotion without ever explaining *why*. The sad reason is that the editorial mention is probably a payoff to an advertiser.

Spending loads of money on cosmetic products is fine if you enjoy it and if it makes you feel better; it's wrong if you're duped. Prestige has its price. But many an inexpensive product will yield comparable results. Unfortunately, in some cases that means none. When you scrutinize the rationale behind recommended grooming procedures, you have clearer guidelines for what products to purchase.

The clothes you wear can be changed daily. Not so your face, body, or hair. A well-groomed fellow looks good in jeans or a tuxedo. An unkempt guy looks good in neither. Despite the saying, clothes don't make the man. Today, when nearly anything goes nearly anywhere nearly all the time, first and foremost is the man, not the color of his socks. Wardrobe is a secondary consideration and is not covered in this book. Fashion changes are often whimsical. You're yourself all your life long. Give yourself some serious thought.

As mentioned earlier, most of us men have been conditioned not to look at ourselves. Now's the time for some shock treatment. Strip and check yourself out in a full-length mirror. Don't suck in your gut; no one's looking but you. Take a good, close look from the soles of your feet (do they have any rough patches?) to the top of your head (you don't have dandruff, do you?). Spend some time reacquainting yourself with yourself. If you're totally happy with what you see, close this book (gently, please) and pass it along to some poor slob who needs it. If you think the door's open for improvement, read on.

Just a few last words before you scan through the remaining pages. Although most men don't do enough to maximize their looks, some go overboard. They can look *too* good, all facade. Or they think they can mask their imperfections. Short of cosmetic surgery, no one can completely make himself over, and even then limitations exist. But there is the manly art of compensation. Carried to extremes, it becomes overcompensation. Trying too hard often shows. Nothing impedes like excess. Someone with "the look" looks real, not plastic. When he plays touch football, he doesn't wear hair spray, but he definitely arms himself with a deodorant.

What is "the look"? I make my living with words,

but I'll be damned if I can describe it. The closest I can come is to say that it's looking put-together, with equal portions of good health and self-confidence yet without looking vain. No, that's not it. It's standing out in a crowd of men by being a better example of what every man in that crowd would like to look like if he had the same raw material. That isn't right either. Is it making the most of what you've got? Yup. It's how you've always wanted to look and secretly felt that you could if you'd try. You can. Try.

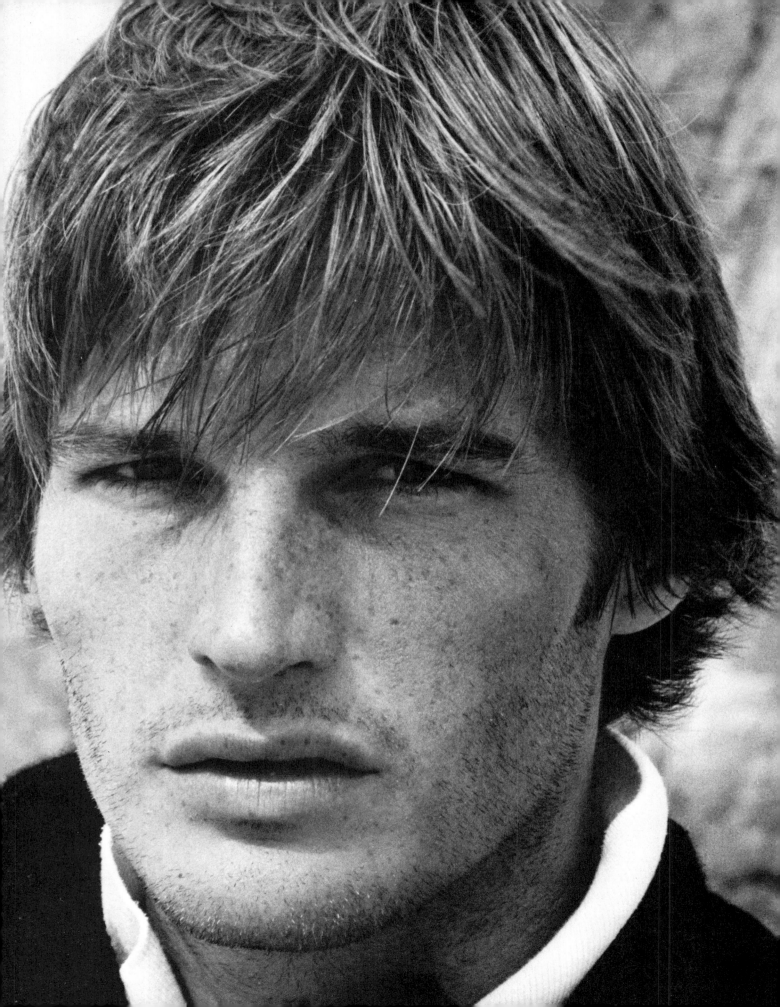

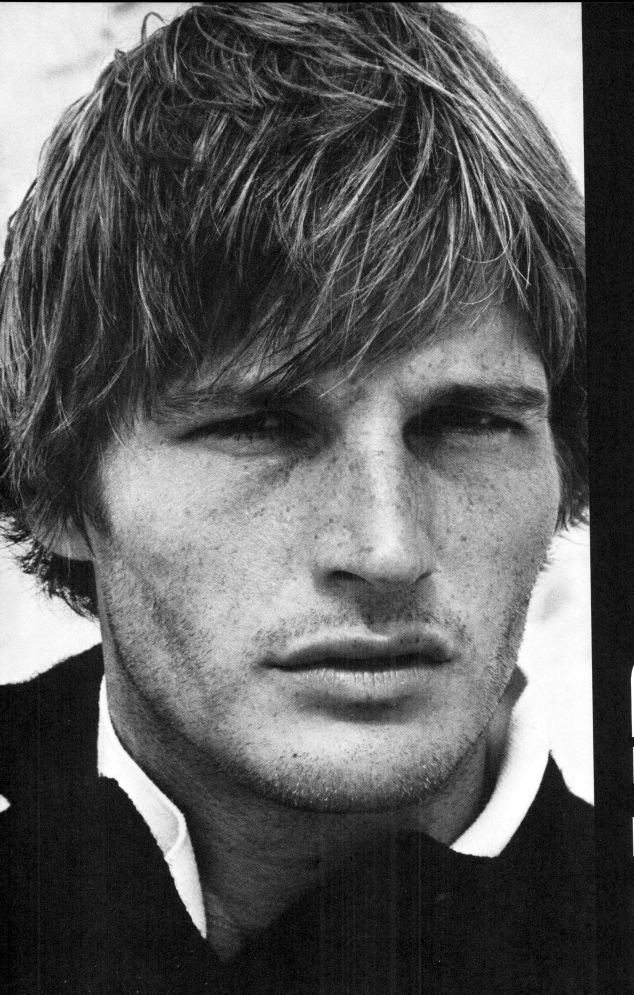

HAIR

CHAPTER 1

MAKING HEADWAY
HAIR & SCALP CARE

Hair is hair. Its needs don't recognize gender. Yet too many men get harried dealing with hair. They consider it their hairiest grooming plight. Is their hair too straight? Too curly? Too blah? they're constantly asking themselves. Should it be shorter? Longer? *Sexier?* Let's be honest. Is hair ever really sexy? Isn't it where your head is at that really counts? Styling quandaries ought to be put into perspective. Far more serious is daily care, since nobody goes to the barber shop every other week any more. If a guy constantly abuses his hair and scalp, he'll have very little to worry about in the not-too-distant future.

VIEW FROM THE TOP
HAIR STRUCTURE

Technical jargon is a bore, right? Who cares that individual strands of hair are called hair shafts or that the hair that we see is dead? Well, if you care about looking good, you should also know some of the facts about yourself and your body. Otherwise you can't determine whether you're helping or harming yourself.

Technical jargon aside, hair is basically a waste product, dead matter eliminated from under the skin. Having no blood supply or nervous system of its own, it must be fed from below and assisted from above. Ill-treated hair weakens, breaks, or falls out.

Every hair strand has a root (beneath the skin's surface) and a shaft (what's visible). The life of the hair all takes place in the root located in a small sac called the follicle. What's most vital for hair growth is the small "bud" at the base of the follicle. This is named the papilla and is nourished by blood circulation. Technically, the papilla is part of the root, although the terms are commonly interchanged. As long as the papilla is alive, hair can grow.

As mentioned, visible hair is waste; it's composed of proteins similar to other body proteins. When new cells are formed within the follicle, the old ones are

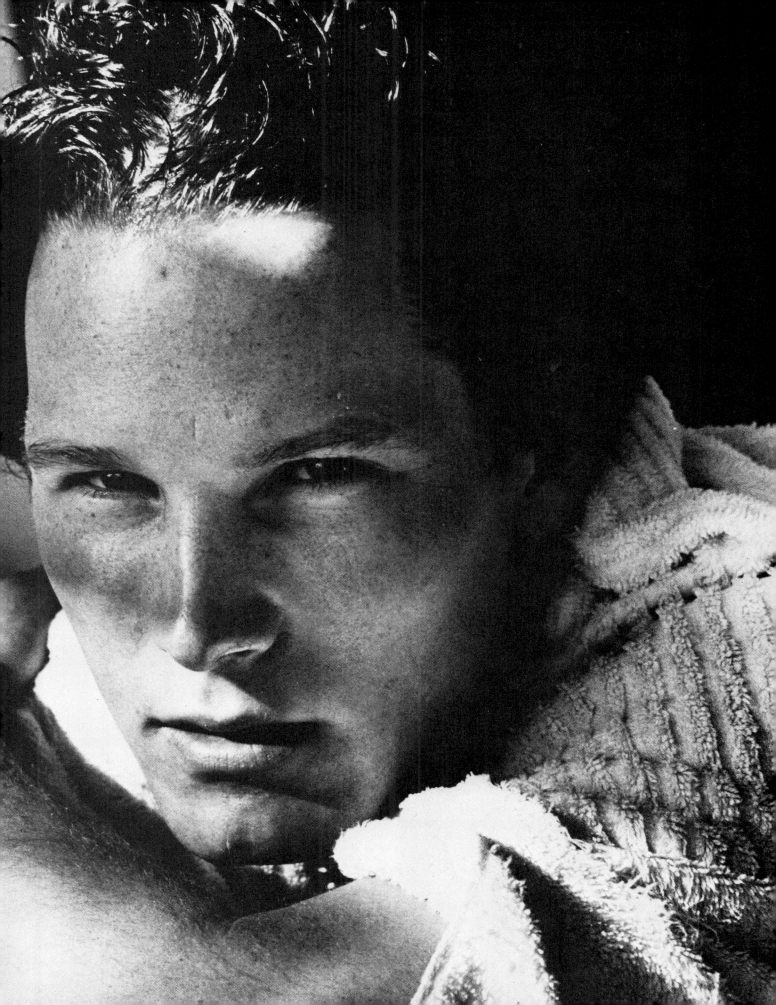

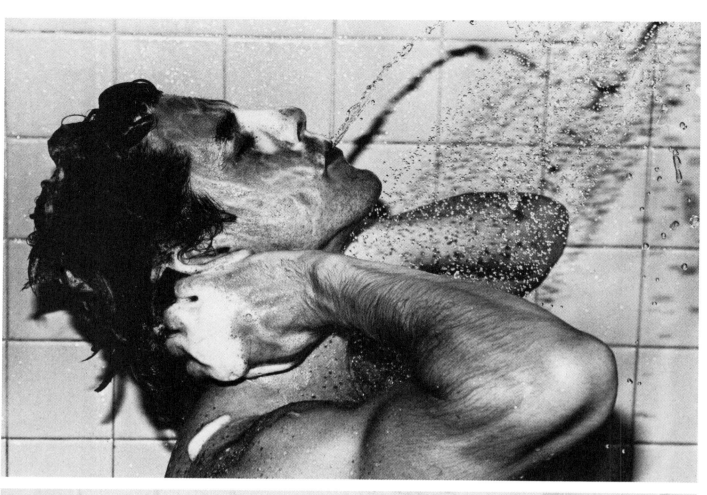

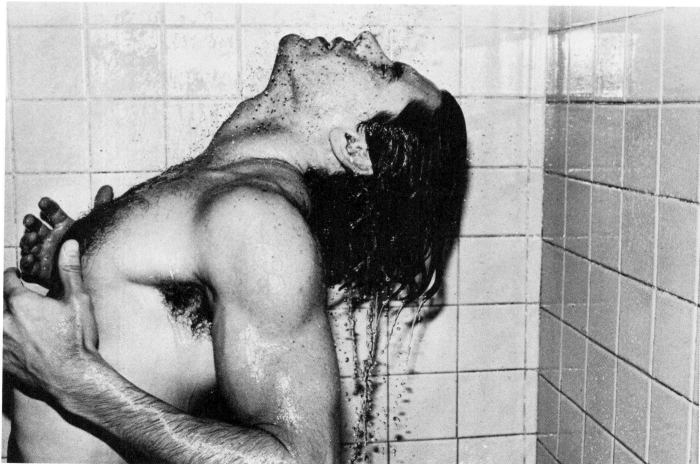

pushed away and up through the pore opening. No longer being nourished, these cells die and become part of the hair shaft.

Residing near every hair follicle are oil-producing glands known as sebaceous glands. Their oil secretions lubricate and protect the hair. When the glands are too hyped up, hair becomes oily. When they're lazy or sluggish, hair becomes dry. When they're nicely balanced, hair is normal. How these glands do their job depends upon age, diet, emotional climate, drugs, blood circulation, and other variables. That's why one's hair condition is not static.

The hair shaft itself is usually composed of three layers: the cuticle (outer) layer, which is protective and made up of overlapping cells that look something akin to fish scales; the cortex (middle) layer that contains color-giving pigment; and the medulla (core), which is little more than a hollow tube and isn't always found in every hair. A missing medulla is inconsequential.

Melanin is the primary pigment accounting for the color of your hair. The pigment is found in small yellow-brown granules; how much and where it's distributed determines hair color. Blonds have small amounts of melanin granules. Red pigment may also be found in the hair. Redheads have little melanin but lots of red pigment. Men with brown or black hair have a combination of both. Fading hair color signifies slower pigment production, while darkening color obviously indicates the reverse. White hair has no pigment. Of course, different hairs have different amounts and combinations of pigments, so no head of hair is all exactly the same shade.

IN A LATHER
SHAMPOOING

Shampooing is the most important step in hair care. Not only the hair, but the scalp also must be scrupulously clean for optimum health and appearance. Although dry or oily conditions won't be cured by shampoos, their effects can be alleviated within reason. A good shampoo adds luster and manageability, imparting a "touch-me" quality. That's as sexy as hair can be.

Shampoos work by dislodging dirt and oils so that they can be rinsed away. But natural protective oils may also be swept away in the process. Therefore, quality shampoos contain conditioning ingredients to supplant some of the removed oils. Harsh shampoos can rob these oils without replacing them.

Many supposed experts belabor the question of how often to shampoo. The only logical answer is, whenever it's dirty. Period. In America's polluted cities, that means daily, unless the hair is seriously damaged. Even shampooing twice a day is fine as long as precautions are taken to offset potential dryness. Oily hair attracts and retains dirt faster and longer, so it requires more frequent shampooing than normal or dry hair.

Everyone knows how to shampoo, right? Wrong.

Ideally, good shampooing begins in advance of wetting the hair. Before stepping into the shower, first give your hair a quick but complete brushing to activate the oil glands and loosen dead scales. Don't overdo; excessive brushing causes irritation. Next gently massage the scalp. Plant the fingertips firmly in place and rotate without slipping against the hairs. If the scalp is tight, more pressure must be exerted. Work from the nape of the neck forward. Give yourself at least one full minute's massage.

Now into the shower. Wet the hair thoroughly. Warm or tepid water is better than hot, since excessive heat shocks the scalp. Add a small amount of shampoo (about one tablespoon) to your palm and lather gently but firmly through the hair. Massage your scalp with your fingertips. The use of a small plastic brush, while considered controversial, can be helpful in massaging the scalp and removing dead cells but only if the bristles are rounded and nonirritating. But if your scalp is sensitive, beware.

Disregard labels advising you to shampoo, rinse, then repeat. Although this is a sure way to increase shampoo consumption, once is definitely enough if you cleanse regularly.

Rinse thoroughly. Many men leave shampoo residue on the hair (which dulls it) and on the scalp (which impairs normal functioning). So after rinsing, rinse again. Then one more time. If leftover shampoo builds up on the scalp, it will eventually flake. This leads some misguided fellows to conclude that they have dandruff (see discussion on page 9).

Before the 1930s, shampoos were virtually nonexistent. Most people washed their hair with body soap. Bad idea. Soap's alkalinity dries hair unmercifully while its hard-to-remove film dulls natural sheen.

Any shampoo on the market will clean the hair, but

there is more—or should be more—to shampooing than cleaning; which brings us to the subject of choosing a shampoo. No easy task.

First, a list of don'ts: *Don't* select a shampoo simply because it smells good; fragrance seldom comprises more than 1 percent of a shampoo's formula and has no effect whatsoever on its cleansing action. *Don't* be misled by claims about superrich lather; foaming compounds are often added merely for appearance's sake. *Don't* expect any shampoo of itself to correct badly damaged hair; none can. *Don't* be taken in by gimmicks; every season brings new shampoo crazes, most of which don't deliver.

The real dilemma in picking a shampoo is the wealth of varieties and brands available. Of the so-called herbal shampoos, some are actually formulated with natural herbs, while others add chemicals to smell "natural." Some reputedly mild baby shampoos are only watered-down adult shampoos; their "mildness" results from the dilution. Organic shampoos boast an array of natural ingredients, hiding the fact that many chemicals, including detergents, are derived from "natural" sources. Nor are protein shampoos instant panaceas. They claim to be compatible with hair (true), since hair is mostly protein, but they can nonetheless contain other harsh or harmful ingredients. Acid-balanced shampoos also claim they're congenial to hair (also true), since their pH factor (degree of acidity) corresponds to that of normal, healthy hair. Yet this is no safeguard against ingredients that might cause allergic reactions.

Of the various types of shampoos just mentioned, some brands are terrific and others are terrific shams. Peering at the bottles can't inform you which is which.

Since shampoos come in preparations for dry, oily, and normal hair, perhaps that should be the primary consideration? Not necessarily.

How often a guy shampoos should affect product choice. If his hair is only moderately oily, for example, and if he shampoos daily with a formulation for oily hair, too much oil may be stripped away: He'd be better served with a normal or even a dry formula. On the other hand, shampooing only once a week with a formula for oily hair would be insufficient for the same fellow. Since daily shampooing is recommended for urban males, only in extraordinary circumstances would every-day use with a formula for oily hair be considered wise. (More about this subject in the "Headaches" section of this chapter.)

Unfortunately, the only way to judge whether a shampoo works for you is to try it. Test a new brand for a week or so. Does your hair have more luster? Is it easier to manage? Is your scalp free of irritation? If you can answer yes to these questions, you've solved your shampooing problems . . . almost.

The sorry truth is that sticking with only one shampoo is a bad idea. Hair builds up a natural resistance to any product constantly used. For best results, alternate between two different brands every several days, never allowing your hair to take you for granted. It sounds idiotic, but your hair will actually look better if you keep it guessing. So, until you discover two spiffy shampoos, keep trying.

TEMPORARY EMPLOYMENT
CONDITIONING

As if shampooing weren't complicated enough, an ongoing debate centers on conditioners.

Conditioners are designed to enhance hair's appearance temporarily, from shampoo to shampoo, by coating the hair shaft, thereby sealing the fishlike scales. Depending on hair health, benefits can be minor (reducing static) or major (restoring softness, shine, and manageability).

Like shampoos, conditioners come in seemingly infinite varieties. *Instant conditioners* applied to damp hair for one to several minutes before being rinsed away coat the hair with deposits to help fill the hair "pores" of the cuticle and make the hair smoother, less likely to tangle. *Body-building conditioners*, sometimes called texturizers, do the same but also add a quantity of fortifiers to increase hair diameter. *Corrective (or therapeutic) conditioners* are usually left on the hair for twenty minutes or more to penetrate more deeply. Supposedly they relieve and prevent dryness, add sheen, restore natural elasticity, and make hair more supple and resistant to damage. Sometimes wearing a heating cap or wrapping the head in a towel is required. Some, but few, conditioners aren't rinsed out. Although the hair may appear improved, it will revert to its original state if conditioning is discontinued.

Another conditioning technique that reputedly improves the hair for a period of time is the *hot oil treatment*. Offered by salons, it can also be self-applied at home. These treatments are primarily for fellows with dry or damaged hair. Often such conditions are accompanied by built-up dead cells on the scalp, which provide an excellent breeding ground for bacteria. The first step in a hot oil treatment is heating a vial of the specially formulated oil by running hot water over it for about five minutes. Using absorbent cotton balls, massage the warm oil into hair and scalp. Comb through to distribute evenly. Then run hot water over a terry towel. Squeeze out excess moisture and wrap the head turban-fashion. Wait ten to twenty minutes, then rinse thoroughly with lukewarm water. Some hot oil products come with built-in mild shampoos, so the hair is simultaneously cleansed. If not, the hair must be shampooed before drying.

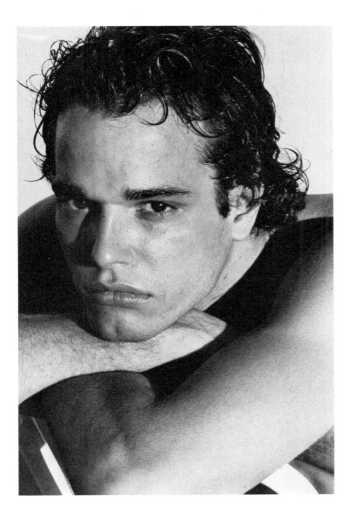

Most hair people agree that conditioning is valuable for dry, brittle, or damaged hair and for men who use blow dryers extensively. However, there is some disagreement as to whether conditioners really prevent minor ills such as split ends or lackluster hair from occurring.

Watching your hair closely is the only way to determine whether or not to use a conditioner. If your hair often tangles after shampooing, such products are definite boons. But if your hair is naturally shiny and manageable, be content. On the other hand, if your hair becomes dull or lifeless from time to time, or if you have split ends or flyaway hair, then you might want to give conditioning a try. With coarse hair, cream rinses (these are actually conditioners) are often the best solution, since they relax and soften. With fine and limp hair, heavy conditioners are literal drags on your hair with unappealing results; balsam conditioners are lighter and milder.

As with shampoos, you can't judge a conditioner unless you try it. Sorry. Bargain brands, however, are seldom bargains.

HOLDING PATTERN
GROOMING AIDS

Hair dressings or tonics, which control unmanageability and dullness, come in tubes, gels, and liquids. Whatever the form, rule number one is to apply sparingly. Overdoing attracts dust and soot, causing the hair to develop the blahs during the day.

Don't be cowed by label instructions. Hair needn't be wet when these products are applied. In fact, you can't even determine the amount you need unless your hair is in its normal state—dry. If your hair looks dull and flyaway, you may at that point decide to use a dressing. When the label indicates that the product should be put on wet hair, dilute the dressing with water in your palm, then gently and evenly work it into your hair.

Freshly shampooed hair that's already been treated with a conditioner seldom needs another dressing. That would add another layer to the conditioner's coating, making the hair sticky and giving it an unnatural sheen.

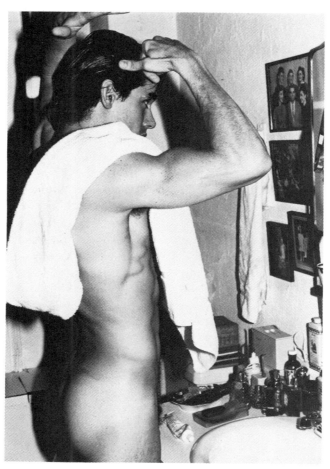

Virtually any type of hair dressing can be used on normal hair. But remember that the first goal of dressings is to keep the hair in place. If you're after the blowing-in-the-wind look, think twice. Also, oils and creams should be applied only to dry, thick hair; for they tend to weight down fine hair too heavily. A gel (an emulsion diluted with water) gives better results. Neither are oils or creams recommended for oily hair; they only aggravate the situation. If a dressing must be used in this case, it should have strong alcoholic content and should be soluble in water.

Ultimately, unless a dressing has a very greasy feel to begin with, evaluation is only possible after trial. (True, this advice was also given for choosing shampoos and conditioners and will be repeated throughout the book. But while experimentation can be a frustrating process, never underestimate the value of trial and error.)

Hair sprays are another way to help keep a style manageable. However, no reputable hair or scalp specialists recommend their use. In addition to the ecological controversy about the effect of aerosols on the atmosphere, heavy spraying can cake the scalp, choke the hair follicle, and retard proper growth.

Spray buildup also increases the likelihood of breakage.

If you must spray, hold the can twelve to fourteen inches from the hair and apply lightly, directing the mist upward toward the hair and not at the scalp. You should shield your eyes with your hand. *Brush out nightly without fail.* Better yet, try one of the manually operated pump sprays: They're cheaper on a cost-per-use basis and are just as effective. Again, avoid overuse. *And brush out before retiring.*

At more expensive price points, there are some nonlacquer hair sprays that are formulated to do more than hold. These sophisticated types, which contain conditioning ingredients, are sprayed on the hair before blow drying as protection against the heat and also to impart luster. Less sticky than the lacquer variety, they offer less control but are healthier. The extra benefits of a more natural appearance may compensate for the higher cost. They can also be used without blow drying, in which case the hair should be toweled dry, sprayed, and then combed into place. When the hair is completely dry, it should be combed again to redistribute the agent and to give more body to the style.

HEADACHES
HAIR PROBLEMS

Genetically, some men's hair is better than others'. Yet weak hair, when cared for properly, can be healthier than strong, good hair that is neglected or abused. No single formula exists for hair care, since many factors, from diet to cleansing to sun exposure, influence hair health. Of course, an unhealthy body cannot produce healthy hair.

Some hair problems are more severe than others. There is even healthy "unhealthy" hair—dry or oily hair that falls within normal confines. Common dandruff is certainly not uncommon. Mild or not, however, it remains a medical problem. Medicated shampoos, if overused, can be extremely hazardous to the scalp. Beware. Mass-distributed dandruff shampoos may check flaking but can also strip the hair of protective oils. If daily shampooing with a mild shampoo doesn't ward off dandruff, see your physician or dermatologist. Even though over-the-counter remedies commonly contain the same or similar ingredients prescribed by professionals—sulfur, selenium sulfide, salicylic acid, zinc pyrithione, and tar—either alone or in various combinations, the choice of lotion or ointment depends on the severity of the condition. Furthermore, in over-the-counter products these proportions cannot be tailored to the sufferer. Nor is there a practiced eye to evaluate their effectiveness and to adjust the concentrations. Another complicating factor is that several types of dandruff exist, ranging from simple (also called dry dandruff), which is characterized by flaking and itching, to severe (also called wet) dandruff, with redness and inflammation combined with itching and flaking of the scalp. The same symptoms may appear on the sides of the nose, around the eyes, even on the chest. The cause of dandruff is unknown, but there is no proof that germs are the primary culprits. Thus, antiseptic shampoos are of questionable value from the outset. Another inherent problem in purchasing over-the-counter remedies is that dandruff can be confused with psoriasis of the scalp or eczema, neither of which respond to formulas to combat dandruff. Thus, there's much danger in self-diagnosis and self-prescription: A man is literally risking his own scalp. Don't.

Improperly cut hair can't look good, but don't be too quick to blame your barber. Some styling problems may be solved by changing your daily hair care regimen. Here are some examples:

Dull, Lifeless Hair

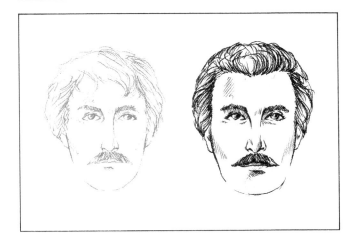

The classic symptoms of dry hair. Investigate conditioners. Simple hair dressings may also work if they don't conflict with your style. Or, maybe your shampoo flunks.

Fine, Flyaway Hair

Usually associated with dry hair. Try any or all of the preceding remedies. Specifically, a texturizing shampoo (a malt type, for example) combined with a body-building conditioner may do it all. When using products to thicken the hair shaft, always quickly brush out nightly to avoid buildup that can make the hair brittle.

Fine & Clinging Hair

Often the result of dry hair but oily scalp. (Yes, this combination can occur.) Treat the problems separately. Use a lotion to counteract the scalp condition but avoid oily shampoo formulas. Instead, shampoo daily with a super-mild variety. Clinging, fine hair might also signal both oily scalp and oily hair. Daily cleansing is again recommended, but with a normal formulation. Although excessive blow drying can harm the hair, careful use can lift the hair and eliminate some of the oily appearance. But never direct the nozzle at the scalp. (See the "Lots of Hot Air" section of Chapter 5.) The heat stimulates oil production.

Greasy Mish-Mash

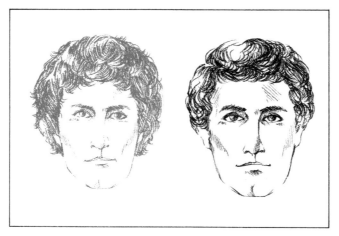

Coarsely textured or dense oily hair often looks a wreck, especially if the hair is longish. Don't resort to hair sprays; you'll look plastic-coated. Cream rinses to relax the hair will worsen the condition by adding more oils. If daily shampooing with a mild or normal formula doesn't eliminate the mess, then cut the mane. Long, oily hair courts complexion crises anyway. Your best solution: clean and short, free and casual, wash and wear.

Spiky Hair

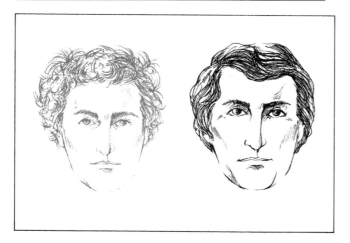

Coarse hair, even when it's otherwise normal, seems to have a mind of its own. If not extra clean, it will sometimes look matted or spiky. Cream rinses to soften the hair may help. If the hair becomes more manageable but looks nondescript after conditioning, consider adding a bit more length. The weight of longer hair tends to keep it in place and adds style.

Damaged Hair

Investigate what you're doing to destroy your hair, then set about healing it. Avoid harsh shampoos; avoid the sun; avoid anything that's hampering. If at-home corrective conditioners fail, rush to a salon for professional hair/scalp treatments. Quick.

LOOSENING UP
SCALP CARE

Because hair can only be as healthy as the skin it grows from, scalp care is integral to hair care. Common to the plethora of scalp-treatment theories—including ultrasonic scalp stimulation—is the value of tip-top cleanliness and good circulation. (As noted, cleanliness is crucial for every grooming zone.)

If the scalp is tight, circulation is sluggish, and hair isn't sufficiently fed by the blood vessels. Keeping the scalp loose, thus improving the flow, is one way to prolong hair fitness. Avoiding stress and anxiety, which really do make you uptight up there, can improve hair's appearance. Easily said. Easily done?

Short of reaching for tranquilizers, another way to stay loose stems from an old wives' tale that apparently works. Stand on your head for a few minutes every day. The idea goes that the force of gravity draws oxygenated blood to your head, stimulating circulation. Similar results can be obtained by lowering the head between the knees while seated, holding the position for several minutes.

Finger massage may be the snappiest way to loosen up. An ideal time is right before shampooing, as stated in the "In a Lather" section of this chapter. Keep fingers firmly in place so as not to tear healthy hair. Don't gouge your scalp with nails, thus risking infection.

Some specialists recommend a minimum of five minutes of daily massage. It can't hurt. In fact, massaging night and morning is not only invigorating but helps in the sloughing of dead cells that comprise the skin's outer layer. If this layer becomes too thick, fresher cells produced lower in the epidermis can't surface. Eventually the hair follicles clog, diminishing hair strength. Preserving the scalp, theoretically at least, should prolong hair life.

While both the scalp and the hair are primarily protein, they are different kinds of protein. Thus, hair products, even those made of the substance, shouldn't indiscriminately be applied to the scalp. That is, hair conditioners are for the hair, not the scalp; ditto for sprays.

Beware the dangers of mechanical abuse. Don't brush overzealously. (Some theorists suggest no brushing ever, a rather extreme view.) Also avoid sharp-toothed combs. Too much hair spray clogs the pores on the scalp. Too strong a stream of hot air from blow dryers can be lethal. In short, treat your scalp gently, lovingly, and tenderly.

Although numerous scalp lotions are sold, especially via the mail, it's impossible to evaluate them all. Each will give a tingling sensation since germicidal ingredients are common to all. Sometimes the tingle may be rather unpleasant. Although not necessarily harmful to the scalp, the sensation may mean that the scalp is overly tight and the pores are bacteria ridden. Diluting the lotion with some water and slowly increasing its strength until the scalp is accustomed to the concentration relieves some of the discomfort.

CHAPTER 2
ALL THE TRIMMINGS
HAIR STYLING

A good cut can't compensate for hair that's in bad condition. But a good style can make healthy hair look even better. Although some cutters tend to play God, ordaining what look is best for a client they've never seen before, this approach seldom works. Since the most common grooming complaint among men is that their hair never looks the way they want it to, obviously a fellow shouldn't be passive in a barber's chair. An honest self-appraisal and a firm resolve are both essential for the man who wants to put his hair style to work. Then he must communicate his desires to a stylist. Alas, the ultimate upper hand is literally the barber's. But a man can always take his hair and patronage elsewhere.

A CUT ABOVE
CHOOSING A STYLE

Generalities about selecting a good hairstyle abound. A man with a perfectly oval face and perfect features, for example, can supposedly wear any style his whims dictate. Taller men reportedly can sport fuller and longer hair than smaller fellows. Square-shaped faces shouldn't carry center parts. All these guidelines are based on the classical rules of harmony and balance. Fine starting points, they don't tell the entire tale.

Choosing a style hinges on one's life-style, age, personality, and career. Currently bushy looks are considered bush league, while well-trimmed is well received. So what? Hairstyle, like clothing style, is personal expression. A man can reasonably go to any lengths he decides . . . as long as he knows in advance what impression he'll make. The California surfer look is great at Laguna Beach but questionable in a corporate hierarchy.

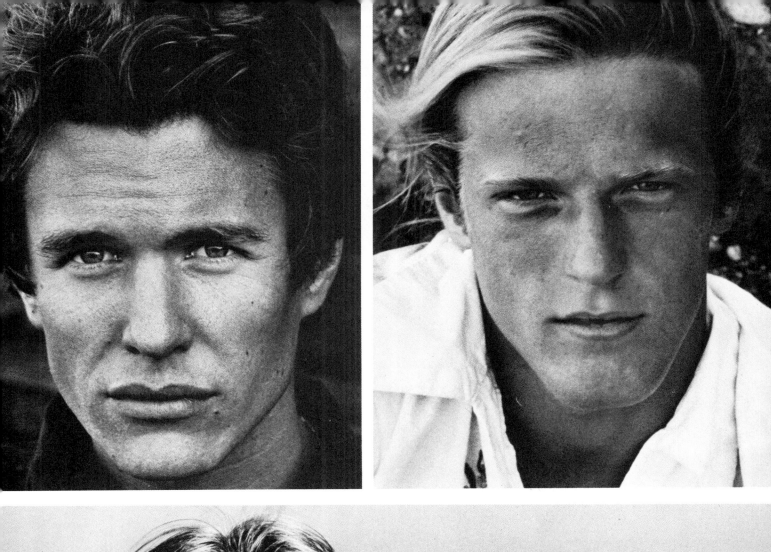
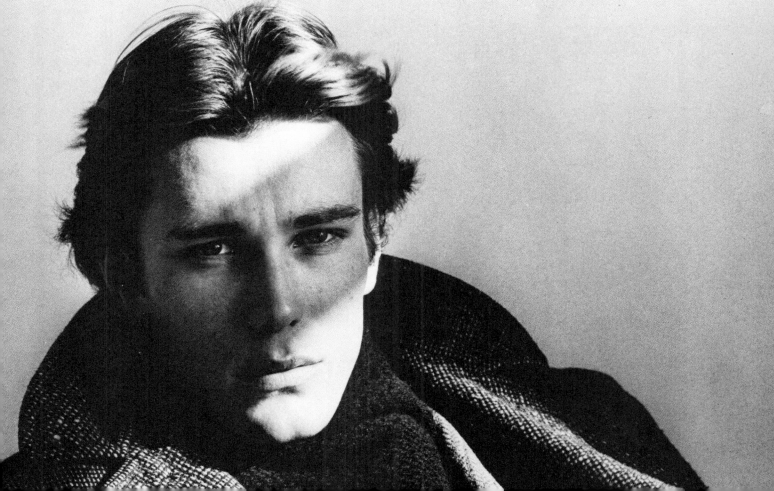

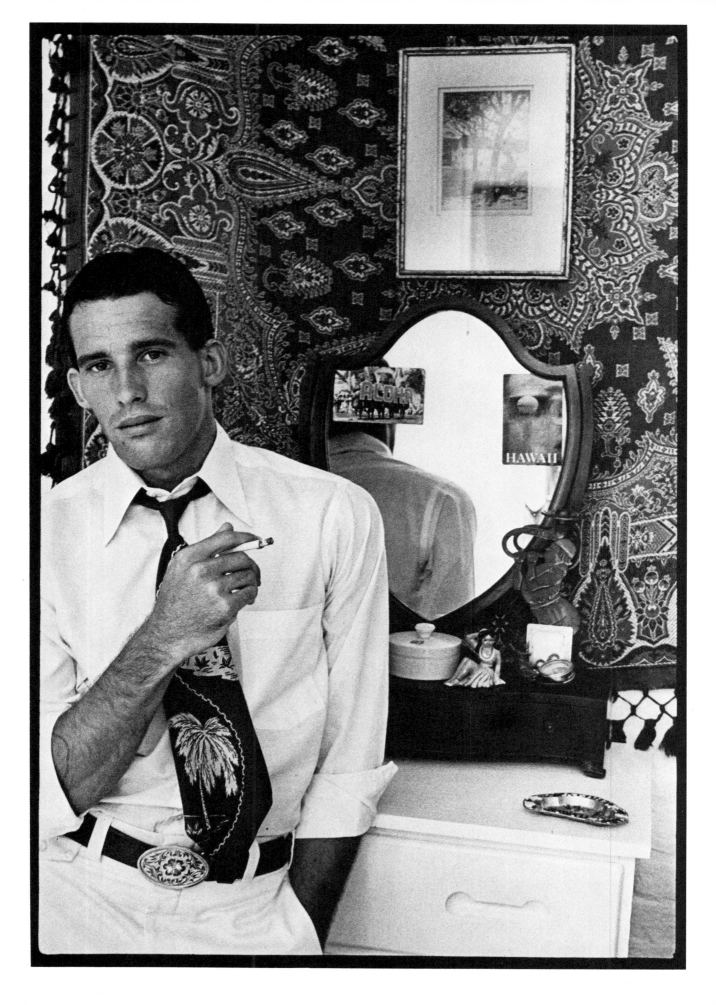

Most men aren't lucky enough to be born with perfect features. Then again, perfection is boring anyway. But imperfections may cross the line from being interesting to distracting. There's a hairline difference between a forehead too low and one with simian ferocity. Large ears that resemble Dumbo's are appealing only to ear fetishists. Angular bone structure can be too sharply severe, not strong. In such instances, it's worth considering whether to put one's hair to work to compensate for demerits. Taking a long, hard look in the mirror to evaluate the individual features is obviously the first step. That old habit of not looking yourself squarely in the mirror must be broken. Here are some points to consider.

Nosing In: The Nose

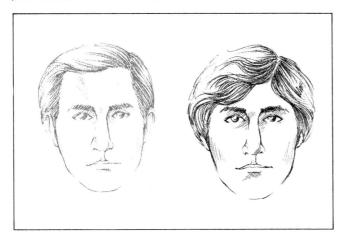

If a nose is very enlarged or awfully underdeveloped, hair length is more important than the cut in redirecting facial focus. So, too, is the decision whether to add a beard and/or moustache. (More about these considerations in Chapter 8, "Fringe Benefits.") Usually when the proboscis is protruding, short hair makes the snout more prominent. Conversely, if the nose is minor, the midface recedes even further with long hair. In both cases, it's advisable to have some hair brushed across the forehead if possible. This adds more diversion. So does a moustache.

Sound Advice: The Ears

A partial solution to ears either too large or too small is the same: Partially hide them. Slicked-back hair a la the greaser fifties is not only outdated but a bad look for anyone who hasn't perfectly proportioned ears. Ear grazing always looks best with a casual and free cut.

To the Fore: The Forehead

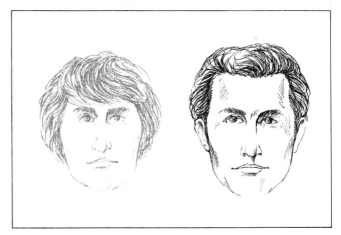

Too high or too low foreheads can be offset by proper styling. Receding hair offers special decisions and is discussed at length in the "Making More with Less" section of Chapter 6. But too low a hairline is potentially more problematical. When there is such low growth, a style should never brush forward on the forehead in bangs or as a hairy vizor. It only accentuates the aspect. Especially on a low forehead, hair shouldn't be too long: A ghoulish aspect results. Perming might help if it won't look as if you're wearing a poorly fitted stretch wig. One straightforward remedy is a side part to divide the hair mass and then combing the hair neatly off the face. If you've the courage, going a bit lighter at the hairline (but carefully, carefully, and performed by a professional, please) makes a vast improvement. (See Chapter 4, "Do or Dye.")

Side by Side: The Sideburns

Men with otherwise great looking hair are often given to weird eccentricities for their sideburns. Why? Are they still caught up in that mystique that hair equals virility, so that wild sideburns should suggest sexual acrobatics? Strange logic. Sideburns should relate to hairstyle. Short hair, short sideburns. Long hair, longer sideburns. But not too long, please. Shaving sharp geometric hedges out of sideburns is bad pruning. Bushy clumps around the ears are just as distracting. To the lobe is as far as any man should go, and that may be stretching it. Sideburn fanciers, take another look. Do you look more masculine or more macho-hung-up? Guys who come on too strong are often those with basic insecurities. Elaborate sideburn treatments can't cover the repressed fears. Get your act together and put those sideburns back into perspective.

The Blahs

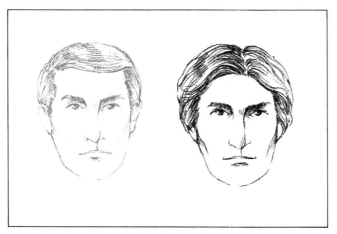

You picture yourself a wizard, but you look more like the cowardly lion. Well, maybe not that drab, but definitely dull. If your features are bland, compounding them with a bland hairstyle will advance the ho-hum impression. Go somewhat more stylized, *not* to extremism, but for more effect. A layered cut, center parted, for extra lift and texture is one of several alternatives. Anything would work better than looking like an anemic bookkeeper.

Berserk

The opposite of a weak-featured face is one with so much strength that the hair must be played down. Yet, if the hair is too short, the strong features might predominate even more. Try a shorter-than-average medium length with no part. Let the hair frame the face but avoid anything rococo or too ornamental.

Perfection

Every hair slicked into submission. Or blown dry to look like a helmet. Face it, the hair is too fastidious and makes you look too vain. Hair she wants to touch is hair you want to have. When your hair looks as if you'll strike should one strand be mussed, it's for ar-

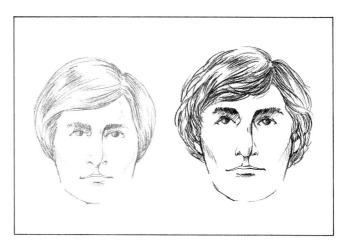

mor not *amour*. Put your hands on your hair and rough it up a bit. Not a lot, but a little. Of course, if you want a stylized Valentino look, okay, but remember that few men—excepting those who live on fashion pages—can carry it off. And when your hair goes ultra, your body must follow. Wardrobe and swagger, even a pencil-thin moustache, may be required.

However . . .

What works in theory doesn't always work in practice. Everyone's hair grows idiosyncratically. Tell a man to brush his hair forward and he'll be the one man in a thousand who has a strange cowlick in the middle of his forehead. Or tell him to grow his hair longer to counterbalance a sizable nose and he'll undoubtedly have very thick, oily hair that goes mishmash past his present length. The condition of the hair—its oiliness, its texture, its density, its manageability—all complicate the choice of hairstyle.

If your hair is extremely oily, it's always better to maintain a shorter style. Otherwise you risk complexion flare-ups. It's no good to compensate with a style that hurts more than it helps. Very fine, wispy hair seldom looks good too long either, because it begins to appear stringy. Thick hair, when not well cut, begins to look bushy after a week or two. Very dry hair, if grown too long, may become brittle, and the ends might split. Very curly hair, too, can lose its shape with extra length. Don't revert to a military look, but if the choice is between shorter and longer, and if your hair isn't tip-top normal and healthy, then the short cut is generally the better route *unless* you're willing to devote extra time and energy to keeping up appearances. With patience and counter-measures, you can do almost anything with hair. It's the true miracle fiber of nature.

CUTTING BARBERS TO SIZE
CHOOSING A STYLIST

Many men can talk to their barbers about everything except their hair. Consequently, they never seem to have their hair styled the way they would like it. The man who has no idea of what he wants must discover a starting point in his negotiations. For openers, how about simply asking, "Do you think my hair is too long? Too short?" The fellow who has only a general idea of what he wants should use conversation to make his desires more specific. It's no crime to be honest. A stylist will be happy to hear, "I like my hair to be easy to care for—I can't hack blow dryers—but I don't look good in short hair; what do you suggest?" Then the cutter knows his client's top priority. The man who knows precisely what he wants must express himself clearly and perhaps face the ire of a prima donna masquerading in barber's clothing. However, any stylist worthy of the name will not be insulted if he or she is presented with a magazine photograph and asked, "Do you think you could style my hair something like this?" But it's wise to remember that hair stylists cut and style hair; they're not plastic surgeons. Maybe they can approximate the style in the photograph, but no stylist can achieve a major overhaul if the basic ingredients aren't there.

One world-famous hair stylist has said, "There's no right hair cut, only wrong ones." A popular psychologist has explained, "One of the few times a man looks closely in a mirror is when he's in the barber's chair. Then he is face-to-face with an image that isn't *him*. He thinks of himself as Mr. America, but the reflection is not someone who looks like Mr. America should. So he blames the barber for what he lacks. Traditionally, the image of the barbershop is of a little boy screaming his head off in the chair. Well, internally, the adult man is still mumbling and still feeling helpless."

So, the foremost consideration in getting the best results from a barber is being honest with yourself. When you're displeased with a certain cut, is it the style or your own looks that you're unhappy with? If it really is the style, don't be Mr. Nice-Guy. Tell the barber, "I don't like it." And be specific. Clearly state, for instance, "My nose looks too big when my hair is brushed straight back."

Conversely, if you like the style, don't just say, "Hey, great!" Sure, it's nice. But if you add, "I really like the way you've tapered the neck," chances are the stylist will more clearly remember how the hair was cut and will duplicate it more easily next go round. For extra security, remind the stylist on your next visit what you liked about the previous cut. Should your instructions be disregarded, you can always cut him down to size: Leave no tip and change barbers.

CHAPTER 3

GOING STRAIGHT, MAKING WAVES
CHEMICAL REACTIONS

For good or ill, many men are ridding themselves of inhibitions governing what they can and cannot do to their hair. Even back in the repressed fifties, it wasn't unusual for a closeted curly-headed male to try to pass for straight by subduing his waves with a chemical straightener. Today, however, males going head-on into techniques that permanently restructure the hair (at least until new growth sprouts) are out in the open and are openly accepted by most. And even if they're not, do you really care?

NOTHING KINKY
STRAIGHTENING

Chemically straightening the hair is akin to perming, only in reverse. The technique is one of unwinding instead of winding. To do so, the chemical bonds of virgin hair (a cosmetics term unimaginatively meaning "untampered with") must be broken down and restructured. During the procedure, the hair becomes swollen and softer, hence weak and more vulnerable. So much for virginity.

As far as formulas are concerned, straighteners are closer to depilatories (see the section on "Rough Go-

ing" in Chapter 12) than they are to perms. If too much tension is placed on the hair while the lotion is at work, the hair simply breaks off; if the lotion is left on too long, the hair literally dissolves. Coarse hair is the safest to straighten. Fine, kinky hair rarely responds properly. Even without hair breakage or loss (both real threats), any hair type can suddenly turn limp and lank if straightening isn't correctly carried to completion.

Since straightening is the harshest, most potentially

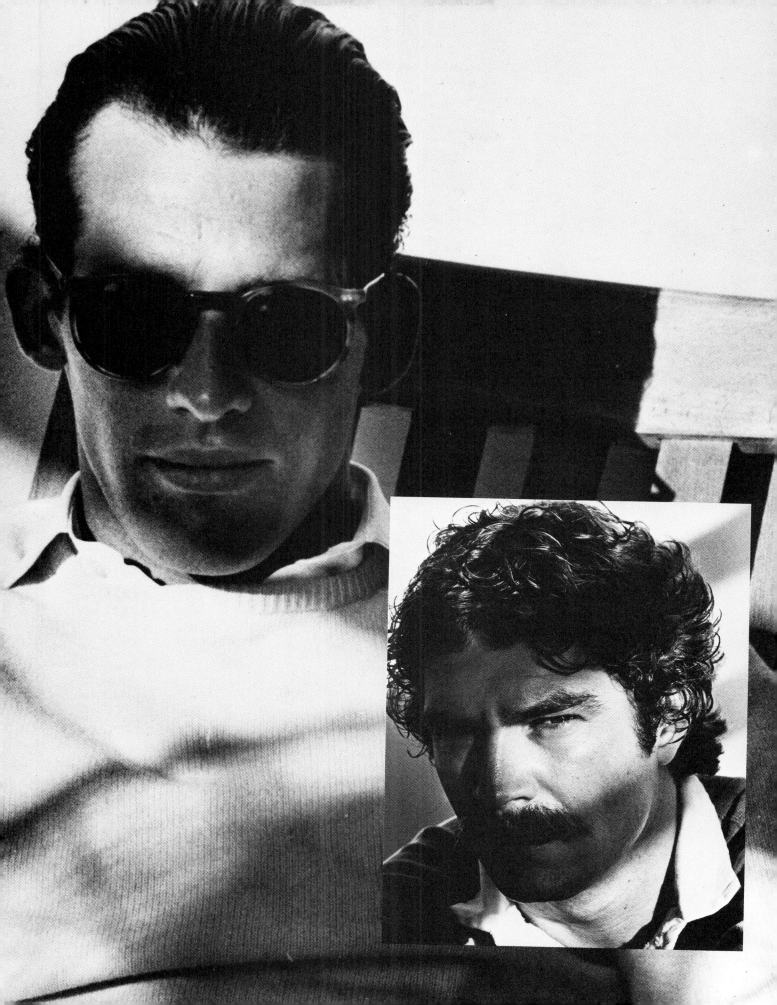

dangerous process performed on the hair, a man should never attempt it himself. Repeat, *never.*

Men who insist upon banning curl from their hair should be forewarned: The process is quite primitive. A protective cream is applied around the hairline and sometimes over the entire scalp, since the chemicals involved in the procedure can irritate the skin. Next, the straightening lotion is combed evenly through the hair, curliest areas first. The hair is—or should be— carefully watched. When the curl is gone, the solution is quickly rinsed out and the hair is neutralized with another lotion. The neutralizer fixes or "rebonds" the hair—that is, the hair molecules are permanently rearranged into a new, straighter molecular structure. Very curly hair can't be made totally wave-free without excessive risk.

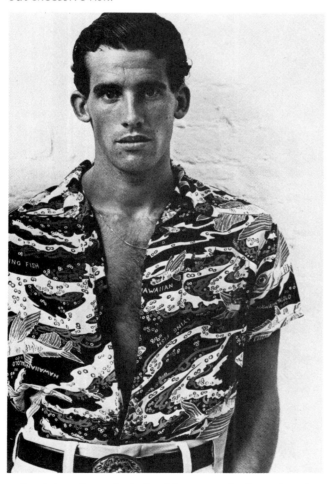

Straightening robs hair of its natural oils and undermines tensile strength. Being more vulnerable, hair then requires extra kindness, extra conditioning, extra *everything,* except exposure to the elements. Too much sun, for example, invites the hair to imitate a haystack.

Pros & Cons

The best thing to be said about chemical straightening is that it is permanent. Shampooing, swimming, and perspiring won't cause uninvited curls to reappear.

Allergic reactions to chemical straighteners are not unusual. Neither are mild (and not-so-mild) scalp irritations.

If hair has recently been colored or otherwise chemically treated, straightening is hazardous. At best, the straightening won't take; at worst, the hair could fall out.

Hair grows about half an inch a month. After straightening, initial regrowth isn't readily apparent, but after a month or two the difference in texture between virgin and straightened hair can look odd. Yet, it is very difficult, indeed next to impossible, to straighten the regrowth without some of the chemicals affecting the previously processed hair and further weakening it.

As straightened hair grows longer, it becomes subject to external abuse. Ends automatically split if precautions aren't taken. Blotting, not rigorously rubbing, the hair dry is especially important considering its weakened state. Occasional hot oil treatments are therapeutic.

When straightened hair becomes too monotonous to care for, the only alternative is to cut away the length that's been chemically treated.

CURL TALK
PERMS

Waving solutions also change the basic structure of the hair shaft. That venerable term *permanent* was well-chosen: Once permed, hair can never be restraightened without risk of severe damage.

Despite the fact that new formulas have been developed to make perms milder and less hazardous, such mildness is relative, since the process still involves harsh chemicals. Home permanents aren't necessarily more or less tricky than the preparations used in salons. In fact, they are often exactly the same. However, do-it-yourself success can be erratically evasive. If directions aren't followed to the letter, disaster may strike. Unfortunately, disasters in professional hands aren't unheard of either.

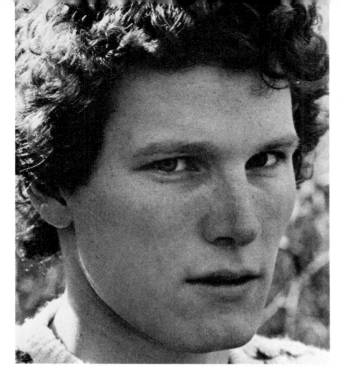

Men may choose perming to achieve various results. For some, the most obvious motivation is the desire to add an abundance of curl. Yet ironically, other fellows purposefully perm to reduce the amount or degree of curly hair, relaxing kinks into waves. This is especially effective on black males; the technique is called Afro perming. Perms can also disguise receding or thinning hair by redistributing curl over the entire head, thereby giving the appearance of more hair. So-called body perms may not add any curl at all; body waving imparts extra lift and control to wispy, fine hair by retexturizing it. Any of these ends are reached via the same basic principle—rebonding the hair into a new shape.

The initial step in a perm, after first shampooing and conditioning, is the application of a lotion to soften the hair. Chemical bonds in the hair itself must be broken down before the configuration of the hair can be permanently changed. This processing step permits the rearrangement of the inner layer of the hair so that it can assume the desired new form.

Next the hair is wound onto rods (curlers), the size of which determines the tightness (or looseness) of the resulting curl. The entire head of hair is again saturated with the processing solution, which remains on the hair for two to twenty minutes, depending upon the formulation. Heat may or may not be required to activate the perming lotion. (Most do-it-yourself and many salon perms are based on the cold-wave concept, meaning that no heat or special apparatus is required.) In some instances, plastic caps are worn to energize the perms. After the prescribed period of time has elapsed, another lotion—the neutralizer—is applied. It counteracts the effects of the perming lotion, reshaping the hair by hardening the new chemical cross-bonds inside the hair shaft to conform to the perming rods. This is the most crucial step. A mistake in timing can cause breakage and hair loss.

Since permed hair has been denatured to some extent, its normal behavior is obviously affected. It tends to dry out more easily, which could make the process desirable for a man with excessively oily hair. As with straightening, coarse hair is permed more easily than fine, limp hair.

When neglected, permed hair can become straw-like. The elements, especially the sun and the sea, more quickly take their toll. On the other hand, when properly cared for, permed hair can be more responsive—with greater body and bounce—than it was before. Since perming is less destructive than straightening or bleaching, normal hair health is more easily regained.

New growth is no great problem with perms, since the new hair is hidden and covered by the processed hair. After two or three months, though, when regrowth can't support the older permed hair adequately, the hair may become rather unruly. Reperming the hair is not especially hazardous, and the previously permed hair can be permed again along with the virgin regrowth. On the other hand, straightening permed hair is far more risky. Thus, the safest way to remove unwanted processed hair is by cutting it off.

Pros & Cons

Unsatisfactory perming results—frizzing, split ends, brittleness, breakage—are usually due to improper processing or neutralizing. Considering how widespread perming is, relatively few serious problems, such as allergic reactions and irreversible hair damage, have been reported in recent years.

Curly styles can be easier to care for, since "finger combing" after shampooing and air drying often finalizes the necessary shaping.

As mentioned, men with oily hair may find their scalp less oily since perming lifts hair from the scalp. Men with fine or weak hair are taking the greater risk with perming. Dry hair becomes even drier, requiring more conditioning and protection from the elements.

The real benefits of perming are cosmetic. If making waves can help you look better or help you think that you do, have no fear: Take the plunge.

CHAPTER 4

DO OR DYE
HAIR COLORING

In any store where hair coloring products are sold, shelf after shelf is filled with preparations for women. If you look very carefully, you may find a meager two or three brands for men. But while women's lines offer at least ten different shades, from Venetian Titian to champagne blonde, for men the selection is usually confined to brown and black. How tintillating. It doesn't really matter if the products being used are created for men or for women. Hair coloring contributes only color. A strand of hair from a man is no different in any way from that of a woman. So, like a woman, a man may choose from a bewildering array of coloring alternatives, even if the packaging isn't geared toward males. At least hair coloring for men—and not only to cover the gray—is no longer behind closed doors.

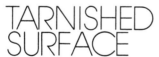

TARNISHED SURFACE
COMB-THROUGH-COLORING

The packages for these often describe the products as hair color restorers. Not true. Since they are exclusively formulated to cover grayness, once the mechanisms of gray are understood, it's clear that comb-through coloring can't restore or bring back a man's own natural color.

Hair color is genetically determined in the same way that skin color is. The more melanin, the darker the color. Although melanin has a yellowish-brownish shade, larger concentrations deposited in the hair can make it appear black. Another pigment, colored red, is also within the hair shaft. But whereas melanin's pigment is fairly solid (or starts life being so), red pigment is, from inception, diffused.

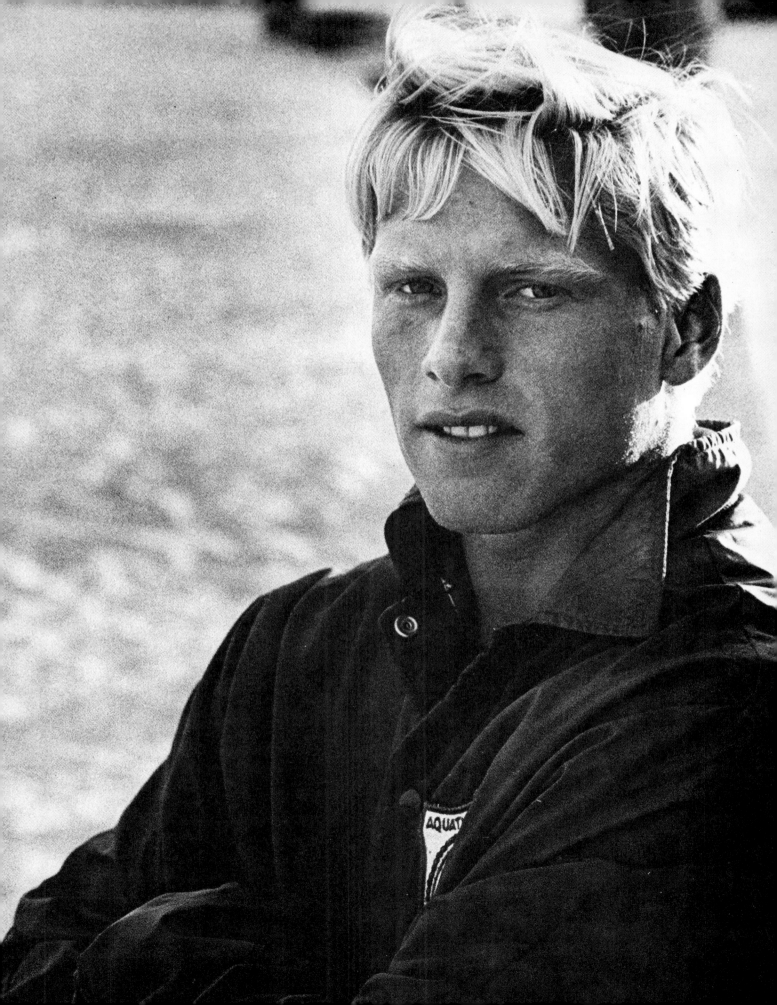

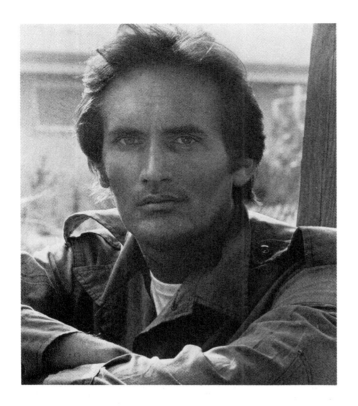

nishing. Hence, there is more discoloring of the hair. All of this occurs on the outer surface of the hair shaft and in no manner creates new pigment.

Since the hair is daily being recoated, natural luster is severely reduced, contributing to a dull and artificial appearance. Shade selection is nonexistent; a yellowish-greenish cast may emerge. The hair may become brittle and susceptible to breakage.

WASH DAY
TEMPORARY COLORING

The name says it all. These coloring agents do not affect the structure of the hair. They merely coat it with harmless dyes that rub or wear off and that can't survive the test of a shampoo.

Usually applied after shampooing while the hair is wet, temporary colorings can be powder, liquid, or spray. They cannot lighten.

When pigment is broken down or when less of it is produced (both the natural consequences of age), more noncolored spaces in the hair create an impression of grayness.

Grayness also occurs when for one reason or another the papilla in the hair follicle stops producing any pigment at all. (This may be related to age or possibly to physical or emotional shock. However, hair can never turn white overnight. In some cases of either shock or illness, pigmented hair may all fall out within a short time span, giving the impression of very sudden grayness.) When isolated hairs no longer produce pigment, as they emerge during growth they are pure white. But other hairs may still be totally or only partially pigmented. The white among the colored and fractionally colored hairs can also bring about an overall appearance of grayness.

Since new pigment production can't be induced naturally within the organism, coloring (not nature's own) must come from external sources.

Comb-through color "restorers" are liquid metallic salts that coat the hair, *dis*coloring it through oxidation. The promoted gradual color restoration really, works as a cumulative chemical reaction. As more of the solution is added onto the hair, more oxidation ensues, a bit like the process of silver progressively tar-

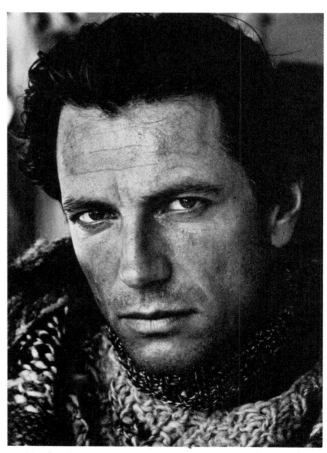

Powder types are dissolved in water, then poured through the hair. By using less than the suggested amount of water, the color becomes more concentrated. The drawback is that the denser solution will likely produce a heavy, artificial appearance.

Liquid rinses often must be mixed with water, too, so the proper color level can be reached. Temporary coloring in the spray form is usually of the "leave-in" variety. It can be messy.

Temporary colorings are often used to cover gray or to make gray handsomer. One subtle method is to apply a temporary coloring (most often called a rinse), which is a shade or two lighter than the natural hair color. For example, if the natural color is dark brown, a medium-brown rinse might be used. Because the natural color won't be affected by the lighter rinse shade but the gray or white hairs will, the overall effect will be a softened hair color without gray.

On the other hand, some men recognize that gray hair can be an asset and want to enhance it, not cover it. Numerous rinses add life and vibrancy to gray by "toning" it. (This technique should not be confused with the toners in double-process permanent coloring, which will be discussed at the end of this chapter.) Gray rinses hide dullish yellow streaks and other unwantables in unattractively gray hair. Avoid the ubiquitous shade used by little old ladies with purple hair in Miami Beach.

The advantage of temporary coloring is obvious. If dissatisfied with the results, a man can shampoo the color away. And therein lies the disadvantage: The color automatically washes away with the next shampoo.

Color on color creates new color. If hair is very yellow and an ash tone is rinsed through, the hair might turn slightly but unmistakably green. Beware.

A SOMETIME THING
SEMIPERMANENT COLORING

This type of coloring falls between temporary and permanent: Like temporary, there's a coating action; like permanent, there's some penetration of the hair shaft. Since semipermanent coloring doesn't alter the natural pigment color or require peroxide, hair can't

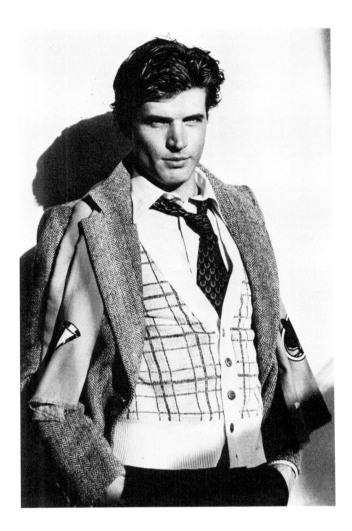

be lightened. Lasting through several shampoos before washing away, this technique blends gray hair into one's natural color, enhances hair that is mostly gray, or deepens an existing drab hair shade.

"Development" time is generally required for semipermanent coloring to take effect. Usually shampooed into freshly cleansed hair, the coloring is worked into a lather that is left on from a few minutes to half an hour, then rinsed away. The longer the development time, the more color imparted. Thus, the same brown semipermanent colorer, for example, can vary in results from light to dark depending upon how long it is developed. Semipermanent colorings have controlled, built-in fading, so reapplication is necessary every few weeks. The frequency of application also affects the depth of color.

The "naturalness" of hair coloring is influenced by color density. In normal hair, shading is uneven. Blank spaces exist in the hair shaft that are without pigment. Light falling upon unpigmented areas simply keeps traveling through until it falls upon a pigmented area and is reflected. However, if too much color (in essence, artificial pigment) is added to the hair shaft, light may be absorbed by it and won't be reflected; the hair looks dead. For this reason, many colorists advise against black shades, since they're more likely to overload the hair with color.

Since melanin colors both the hair and the skin, the normal aging process brings gray hair as well as a sallow skin tone, for pigment is being destroyed or produced more slowly. When covering gray, some men attempt to recapture the hair shade of their teens or early twenties. A mistake. Hair color will contrast too strongly with skin tone and draw attention to itself, a dead giveaway. Generally, as people grow older, their hair should be colored lighter, not darker. And who wants to be a teenybopper anyway?

LIGHTWEIGHT
"LIFTERS"

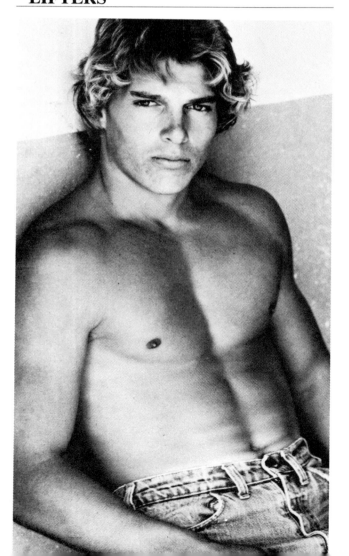

By definition, these colorers (also called mild lighteners) should be considered in the permanent-coloring category, since their slight lightening can't be shampooed away. However, lifters contain so little bleach that they only lighten hair by one to three shades and with minimal damage. Considering that there are numerous shades of blond alone, a shade or two is very little, just enough to brighten drab hair without drastically altering the color. The effect is undetectably similar to natural bleaching from sunlight, except the results are more even and less drying to the hair. One coloring company doesn't call its lifter a colorer at all. The firm describes it as a conditioner, since extra goodies are formulated into the product.

ALL THE WAY
PERMANENT COLORING (SINGLE PROCESS)

Permanent colorings penetrate the hair shaft and chemically alter the pigment. The resulting color cannot be shampooed away; it remains until the hair grows out and is cut off. The root hair may require retouching as it grows.

The term *single process* is a technical distinction and sometimes a confusing one. Basically, it means that the agent colors all of the hair to its desired shade at the same time without any additional step. Application is frequently performed by shampooing or foaming in the tint. However, in some instances, the hair dye must be mixed with an equal volume of developer (peroxide) immediately before using. The dyes are inert until activated by the developer. When mixed and applied to the hair, a chemical reaction takes place within the shaft to produce new color. Obviously, since the new color is formed from within and is not a coating, the results are permanent. If someone is unhappy with the results, the color can only be altered with difficulty and hazard.

Single-process colorings can lighten hair slightly, some more so than others. But none can change a dark brunette into a pale blond without prebleaching (the first step in double-process hair coloring).

With one-step permanent hair colorings, the natural hair color affects the outcome. For example, on red hair shampooing in a shade called natural pale ash blond will probably result in a strawberry blond, but on dark brown hair the action may result in a lighter

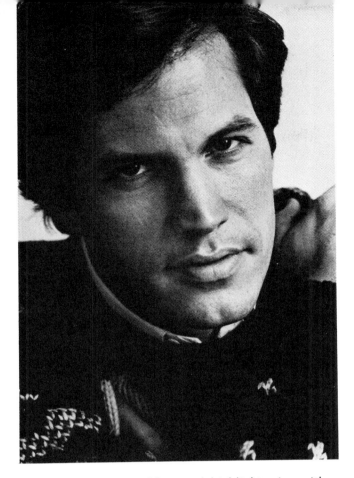

TAKE IT ALL OFF
PERMANENT COLORING (DOUBLE PROCESS)

Two-step colorings produce more dramatic changes, always incorporating some lightening and usually lots of it. The first step is bleaching the hair to remove enough of the natural color so that a secondary dye (the toner) can be applied later to achieve the exact shade desired. Going from black to pale blond is not recommended, since the prelightened hair must be as pale or paler than the toner shade selected. Such a drastic change assaults the hair unmercifully. Not only does prebleaching (with ammoniacal hydrogen peroxide) remove color, it must also make the hair more porous so that it can receive and hold the toner. Timing is crucial, since the hair's natural resilience and strength are being undermined.

Although hair can be severely damaged if the bleaching stage is not properly executed, only the processed hair will be affected. Regrowth will happily be healthy.

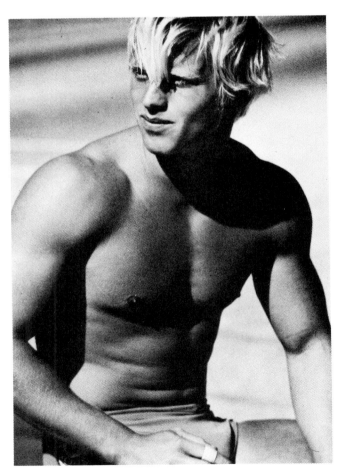

brown with some gold or red highlights. In neither case is a pale ash blond hair color likely.

Redness is a source of misconception about hair coloring. Unappealing reddish highlights often accompany bad coloring jobs. Hair is lightened, whether slightly or extensively, by removing an amount of pigment in the shaft. The more pigment destroyed, the lighter the hair. As mentioned earlier, brown pigment is often a fairly solid mass and is thus more easily assaulted. But red pigment, diffused in smaller deposits, is more evasive, so it may survive longer than brown pigment simply because it's not a sitting target. Lightening hair, then, doesn't add red, but that hue may be uncovered merely by ridding more of the brown. This is only one reason permanent hair coloring is usually not recommended as a do-it-yourself project. The results for the inexperienced aren't easy to gauge. In order to validate uniformity of color, manufacturers photograph for their packaging only models whose hair has been stripped to white, then colored with the same formulated dye as you'll find inside the package. Thus, the hair color on the package will be faithful to what's inside, but not necessarily faithful to the actual results. Darker shades, though, are usually more reliable, since lightening isn't involved.

HALF MEASURES
SELECTIVE COLORING

Various techniques permanently color only pre-determined portions of the hair, not all of it. *Color weaving*, for example, is a technique of enhancing drab hair by brightening more than lightening. The hair is examined for natural light accents. Then individual hair strands are separated by a comb to be treated by two or three different lightening shades. On brown hair the tints are in the bronze/gold family. Paintbrush application further controls the subtle changes. As only a small percentage of hair is permanently colored, the regrowth pattern isn't jarring. *Framing* (lightening only at the hairline), *frosting* (a two-step operation that prelightens, then tones selected strands), *streaking* (placing color strategically in one, two, or several linear locations), and *tipping* (lightening and toning only the ends of the hair) are other examples of selective coloring. With the exception of color weaving, which can yield very natural-looking results, most selective-coloring techniques are probably too extreme for most men.

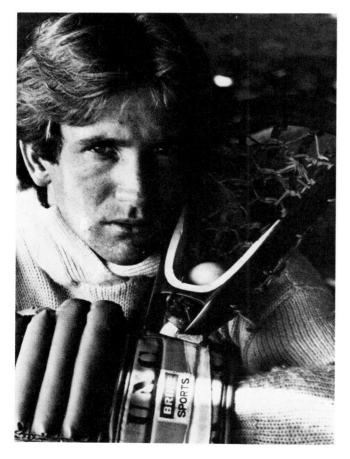

SALAD DAYS
VEGETABLE DYES

Although vegetable dyes predate chemical hair coloring by centuries, henna is the only one still used with any prevalence. An organic conditioner, henna also stains the outer layer of the hair. Standard henna, which is derived from dried, ground-up leaves and stems of a shrub indigenous to North Africa and the Near East, imparts a reddish or auburn tone, while bronze henna produces more golden highlights.

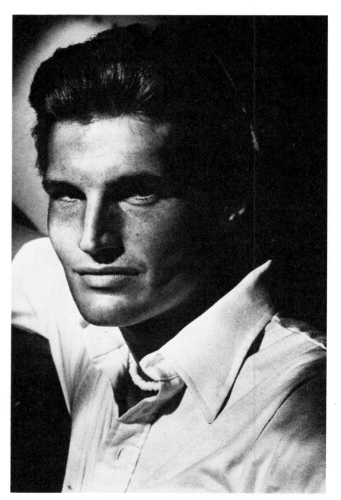

The powder is mixed with hot water to form a thick paste, then brushed into the hair. Since henna works on a heat principle, a fellow usually sits under a heat lamp. The amount of exposure to the heat determines the amount of color change. Since henna fades with time, reapplication for regrowth is seldom necessary unless someone wants to maintain the color.

Coloring Pros & Cons

Any man considering coloring must accept the premise that from the standpoint of healthy hair, it's not the best thing to do. Truthfully, it's purely a cosmetic consideration. On the other hand, coloring doesn't necessarily hurt the hair. Temporary rinses, which disappear after the first shampoo, if not in a swimming pool or on a towel, are harmless if not helpful. Comb-through coloring may make the hair brittle, but proper conditioning works preventively. Unhappily, conditioning can further distort the already questionable color. Even with semipermanent and permanent coloring, properly cared-for hair can remain healthy, usually despite, not because of, the coloring. However, fine, very thin hair may have more body and can become more manageable after coloring. Surprisingly, thick and oily hair can become both softer (since the coarse hair is weakened) and less oily (because of the drying qualities inherent in coloring). Normal hair will become slightly less soft and will be given to dryness, which any decent shampoo and conditioner can counteract.

Once the decision to color the hair has been made, the question arises whether it should be done at home or done professionally. The answer hinges on self-confidence and guts. Presumably salon colorists are more adept than the man on the street. If someone wants to risk his own hair at his own hands, the best advice is: *read*. Read the package, read the label, read the instructions. Improvising is improvident. If a mistake happens, professional help is imperative. Don't experiment. Follow the directions religiously.

Whenever the coloring is performed, a patch test is essential. It probes for hypersensitivity or allergic reactions. The simple procedure involves applying the colorer (mixed as for actual use) to a patch of skin, either at the neck, behind the ear, or at the inner elbow, leaving the tested area untouched for twenty-four hours. Any abnormal reaction, such as inflammation or a rash, indicates that this particular formula can't be safely used by this particular person. However, a patch test should be repeated prior to every coloring, since allergic reactions are often spontaneous.

Also highly recommended, especially if the coloring is self-executed, is a strand test to preview the color. A small swatch of hair is snipped off, the colorer is applied to it. This will help determine the exact time needed for desired results. It can also prevent a catastrophe if the resulting color is horrendous.

The most tedious aspect of coloring is touching-up the roots. Fortunately, some techniques require none. Temporary rinses don't, since new color must be totally reapplied following every shampoo. Semipermanent coloring is generally of the shampoo-in type, so that's no problem. Most single-process permanent colorings are nondrastic, so the entire head of hair can be recolored every several weeks without a noticeable difference between the roots and the previously colored hair. In selective coloring, since only a percentage of the total hair mass is actually changed, the roots tend to blend into the noncolored hair.

Double-process coloring, which always demands prelightening, also always demands root touch-ups. The difficulty is to avoid the previously colored hair. During touch-ups, the coloring agent must also process the virgin roots for precisely the same time as the original job. If the dyes overlap or are processed for different times, the root will be one color, the older hair another. As overlapping touch-ups progress, more bands of different colors will appear on the hair shafts. No good. The touch-up problem is a good argument for having dramatic color changes performed only by pros. Or for not undergoing dramatic color changes to begin with.

Besides the touch-up dilemma, a severe color change increases the risk of allergic reaction and of damage to the hair. It also flirts with potential dryness, brittleness, and breakage.

Permanent hair coloring should never be done more frequently than every four weeks, since the hair can become too fragile.

Despite all these warnings, hair coloring has a definite role in looking good. Blaring color is offensive on females as well as on males. Subtlety is the best guideline not because hair coloring is shameful but because flamboyant hair coloring looks a crying shame. Color weaving, though the process is time-consuming, offers great potential for males who want their hair to look more alive but who can't get it that way using nonchemical means.

CHAPTER 5
TOOLING AROUND
HAIR IMPLEMENTS

A barber's magic can seemingly be dispelled by one night's sleep and one morning's shampoo. Even minimum-maintenance wash 'n' wear styles are more myth than reality. In theory, properly cut and healthy hair should always look tip-top. But hair is often cut defensively to counteract unusual growth patterns. To complete the style, the hair is then blown dry in professional establishments. Since heat relaxes the hair, it assumes a different shape than if air dried. Airflow directions also mold hair diversely. Even when not blown dry, the outcome will depend upon how the hair is combed while wet. These variables explain why one's hairstyle doesn't always look the same. Add varying weather conditions—wind ruffling the hair, humidity frizzing it, cold constricting it—and it's clear that hair implements of some kind, even fingers, are often necessary to keep the hair in optimum shape. The tools employed affect the outcome.

LOTS OF HOT AIR
DRYERS

In the bygone days of the crew cut, all a guy needed was a brush. When the ducktail gave matrons palpitations, a jar of gunk and a rattail comb sufficed. But with today's freer, more liberated men's hairstyles, dryers are often essential not so much to dry the hair as to maintain a desired look.

Actually, the least damaging way to dry hair after shampooing is by gently blotting out excess water with a towel (since hair is its most vulnerable when wet, furious rubbing may rip and tear it), then letting nature take its course. Going outside with wet hair not only courts a cold, it also ensures that hair will dry

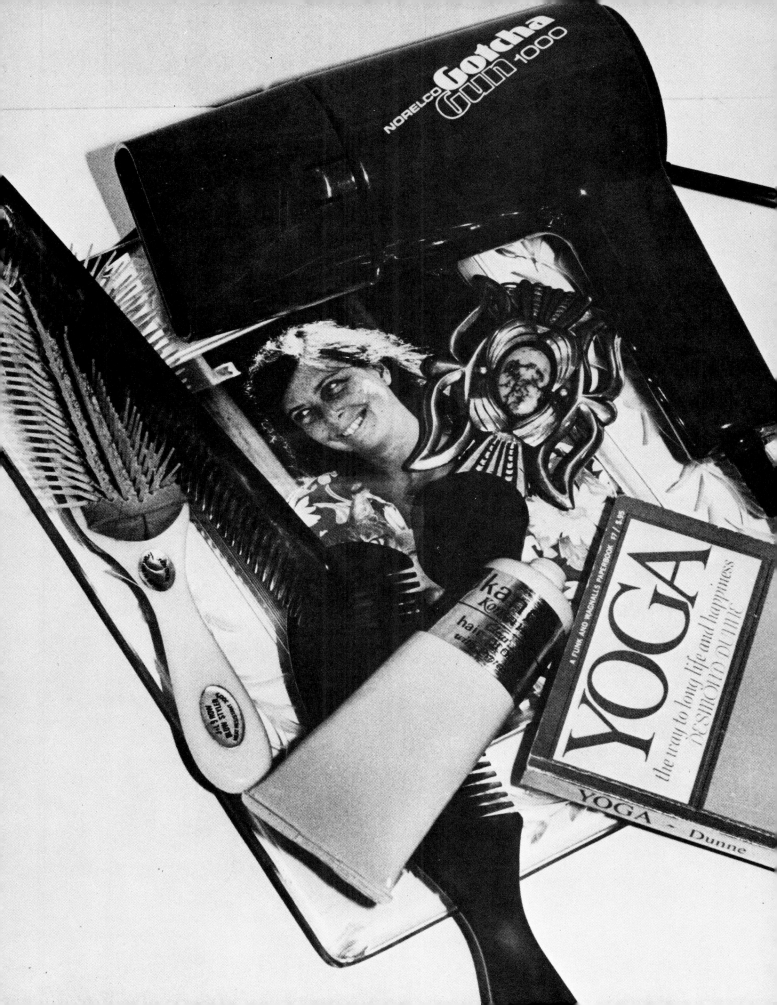

into Mixmaster dishevelment. Dryers, then, are often a necessity.

Although terminology varies, two types of dryers are widely used by men: styling dryers (also called styler-dryers) and professional dryers (also called blow dryers, pistol-grip dryers, pro guns, and assorted other names).

Styling dryers, whatever their shape, are always self-contained units designed to be held in one hand, with styling attachments (combs, brushes, and so on) for clipping onto the apparatus.

Professional dryers, the same as those used by hair stylists, differ in that brushes and combs are *not* attachable to the unit. Instead, one hand aims the blower's airflow toward the hair while the other manipulates a styling tool until everything's in place.

Since some dryers can literally fry an egg, they can harm the hair if misused. Men who are susceptible to dry scalp or dandruff should be especially careful when relying on them. These fellows should take the extra time to dry on lower settings, which remove less moisture from the scalp. Similarly, but for different reasons, if the scalp is oily, only lower settings should be employed, since too much heat can activate oil-carrying perspiration. Fellows with normal scalps and hair, if they're sane in how they dry and style, needn't worry. The airflow should only be directed over and through the hair, never toward the scalp. Extra conditioning or sprays created expressly to add a protective coating prior to drying do help prevent mechanical abuse.

Styling Dryers

Initially, these models seem easier to use than professional types because they're operated like over-sized combs or brushes. In fact, the attachments (plastic or bristle brushes, plastic combs, detanglers, and others) are affixed directly atop the encased motor. There is generally less styling versatility than with the professional versions. Drying efficiency is similar. It's recommended that the attachments not be used during the initial drying stage, until most of the moisture is dissipated. Then flick the temperature and airflow gauges to a lower setting and complete the style, using the desired attachment. Most advanced styling dryers have three switch positions: off, style, and dry. Obviously, the first turns the device on and off. The dry setting combines maximum heat and

air speed to hasten water evaporation from the hair. The style setting reduces heat and moderates the air velocity so the hair doesn't blow wildly while you're trying to subdue it into place. For curly hair, the style setting is often superfluous, since holding the unit about a foot from the head until all the wetness is removed, then simply shaping with the fingers, usually suffices.

Advertisements place too much emphasis on dryer wattage. What really matters is the combination of heat and airflow, which has more to do with engineering than with wattage. And while there is an appreciable difference between 500 and 1,000 watts (*if* the hair is very long and/or thick) in the amount of time you save, the distinction between 750-watt models and those with 650 is negligible. Furthermore, a 500-watt dryer isn't a weakling for someone with normal-length hair.

Although the number and type of attachments vary by make and model, any combination of the following might be included with a styling dryer.

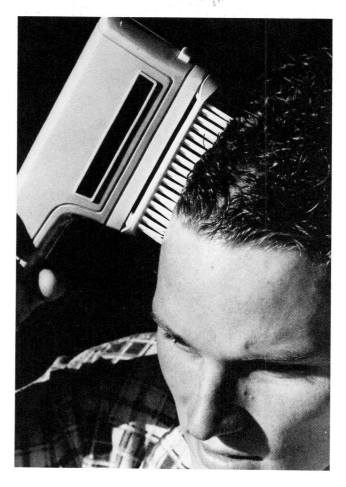

Detangler: Either a comb with two sets of teeth that vibrate to detangle long hair or a comb with one row of widely spaced teeth that separate and lift thick hair to augment drying.

Styling comb: Usually having finer teeth, it is used when hair is nearly dry to provide shape and fullness for thin or fine hair.

Teasing comb: Serrated, or toothed, combs give additional bulk when hair is lifted and combed toward the scalp.

Brush: Contoured bristles distribute the hair and shape or straighten it, especially when hair is brushed from underneath and in the opposite direction from that of normal growth.

Spot dryer: A nozzle directs a concentrated airflow to overpower stubborn wisps, ends, or cowlicks.

"Misters" aren't attachments but built-in devices that spritz water to relax unruly hair so that it can be dried into place.

All manufacturers include use and care instruction booklets, although information is always on the sparse side. Step-by-step, photo-by-photo procedures are seldom found. So experiment with different techniques. What at first feels clumsy becomes second nature over a period of time. Your hair stylist, too, may be able to give valuable instruction for your particular style. Don't hesitate to ask for it.

When using styling dryers, don't daydream. If you idly direct too much heat and airflow onto any one area, you may blow that section into a difficult-to-manage mess. Keep the unit moving, following the direction of hair growth, since good hair stylists usually cut hair according to natural growth patterns. Go against the grain only to impart extra fullness (beware—on males the bouffant look can become the buffoon look) or to wrestle down cowlicks. If you must force your hair, be gentle.

Although every manufacturer of hair implements insists that potential hazards are minimal, all advise against dryers being used by children. That means they're not adult toys either.

Professional Dryers

If you want your hair to look professional, shouldn't you use what the professionals use?

So reasoning, some men feel compelled to buy pistol-grip units. Sorry, fellas, but by yourself you can never get the physical leverage that a stylist has. Also, unfortunately, hair stylists use these high-powered models for speed as well as for style. Since a cutter's take-home depends on turnover, he or she wants to clip right along. Professional dryers with high wattage and concentrated airflow are fastest. For at-home use, mini models may take you a bit longer, but you might find them more manageable. Unfortunately, some lightweight sizes with turbo-type shapes requiring a small DC motor will also have a shorter life-span.

Some men are intimidated by the manual dexterity required to use professional dryers well. They feel awkward the first several times, but practice, if it doesn't make perfect, certainly improves the results. If a man is right-handed, he should grip the dryer in his left hand, keeping the nozzle several inches from the head and directing the airflow upward and through the hair, not toward the scalp. Since styling brushes aren't attached, there's more flexibility with a professional dryer. The nozzle can be directed precisely, and the unattached brush, usually a half-round or circular styling type, is held in the other hand and is manipulated more freely. The brushing accessories must be purchased separately.

As with styling dryers, the first step is to remove most of the wetness from the hair after a gentle toweling. In addition to on/off, most advanced models have two speed settings and two, three, or four heat settings. For someone with normal hair, the initial drying can be done at highest speed and heat. For the final styling, these settings are reduced.

To eliminate unruly hair nuisances such as cowlicks or patches that spike/curl up at the collar, use a natural-bristle or a combination natural/synthetic brush, since heat can warp pure nylon or plastic. Starting at the base of the problem area, spin the brush in the direction you want the hair to lie once it yields its flip. Rotate the dryer from side to side to avoid singeing.

Most blow dryers come with concentrator heads that affix to the nozzle of the unit. These maximize heat and airflow to weaken stubborn hair's resistance and force it into a shape it naturally resists. At these increased heat settings, error can mean tribulations for hair health. And the skin can be scorched. Try to keep the nozzle pointed up and over—not down and into the hair and scalp. And keep the unit in constant motion.

Extremely curly or very thin hair can't always be

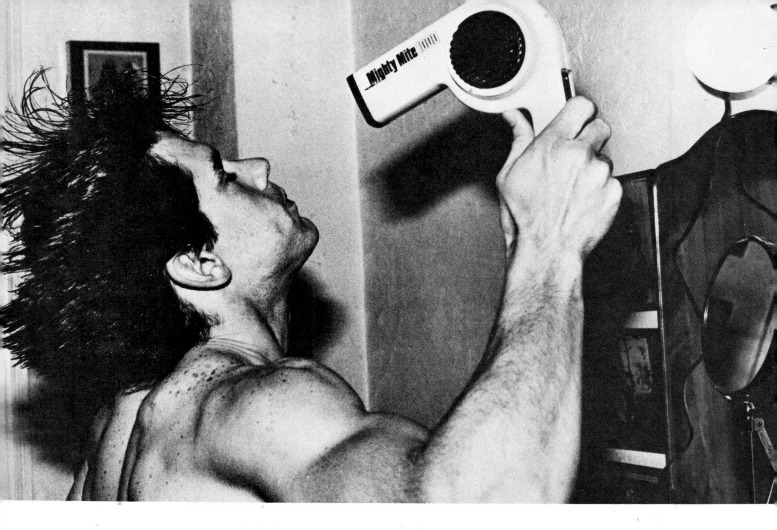

blown dry into a flattering style. Often the hair ends up looking flyaway.

The informational brochures created by manufacturers are only so-so. Personal experience and experimentation will soon serve the user far better.

TOOTHSOME GUIDES
COMBS

Despite some professionals' advice that the only proper comb is one of tortoiseshell—an endangered species—there's little evidence that a well-designed plastic or nylon comb isn't just as functional. The comb's primary role is to arrange the hair properly while lifting slightly, without tearing or pulling, to impart fullness. A comb's teeth should never be sharp or scratchy.

A rule of thumb for testing the comfort and efficiency of a comb is to run your thumbnail very quickly but firmly along the row of teeth. If your nail doesn't glide smoothly along or if it becomes scraped, the teeth are not smooth enough. Since your hair is far more delicate than a fingernail, the sharp edges or nicks in a bad comb will snag in the scalelike outer surface of damp or even dry hair.

Combs should also have some "give" or "play." The reason? The old irresistible-force-versus-an-immovable-object theory. Try as you will, snags or knots have ways of reappearing. When a comb encounters them, if the teeth don't allow some give, your scalp can become bruised or your hair torn. That is why metal combs have especially dubious value: They can wound like bayonets.

Vulnerable wet hair should be combed with care and patience. A wide-toothed comb is the only type recommended at that time. For use throughout the day, a finer-toothed comb is preferable and will give hair a smooth, finished appearance without matting it down the way a brush can. Regular combing not only trains the hair into its style and makes it appear fuller but removes a certain amount of dust, dirt, and airborne debris as well.

Don't dig. Even comb teeth that aren't sharp can damage the scalp. Comb the hair, not the head.

One recommendation that almost no one ever follows: Clean your combs whenever you shampoo. What good is cleaning the hair if you immediately put dirt and bacteria back into it? Keeping tools clean is especially important for men with oily scalps. The more oil on the hair, the more oil that rubs off on the comb, causing the comb to attract more pollution. Soaking combs in dishwashing detergent and rinsing them first with water and then with an antiseptic mouthwash does a good and thorough job. If this method seems primitive, you can always swish some shampoo in a small amount of water and drop your combs into the mixture. Rinse under tap water and let dry on a terry towel or upright in a glass.

BOARING
BRUSHES

Natural boar-bristle brushes—very compatible with hair—enjoy a certain snob appeal. The bristles are deliberately drawn to different lengths to produce an uneven surface so that the scalp can be massaged and stimulated without irritation. Reputedly, these bristles, which come from the back of the wild boar, cannot break or split and thus shouldn't snag.

Contrary to popular belief, however, brushing is of limited value in styling, unless a specially designed, curved styling brush is used in conjunction with a blow dryer to force hair into a specific shape. Without the lift that accompanies the blower's hot air, brushing alone may cause a flattened—even a matted—look.

The main purpose of brushing is to redistribute natural oils evenly along the hair shaft. Countering those who swear by brushing are a growing number who suggest that one hundred strokes are for self-destructive folks. Years ago, when people tended to shampoo only once a week or so, brushing would rid hair of some excess dirt and oily buildup. But today many critics believe that brushing is only psychologically

soothing. Overbrushing by men with oily scalps is thought to increase the oil production.

Whether your hair benefits from brushing, then, depends upon cleansing practices and how much oil is secreted on your scalp. If both scalp and hair are dry, regular brushing may help the hair appear more lustrous, but overzealous action is to be avoided. Dry hair is less supple and more easily broken. For this reason, many hair stylists recommend Denman-type brushes—those with rubber cushions into which bristles (natural or synthetic or a combination of both) are set, allowing for more give and less pull to the scalp and hair—as the most gentle brush for anyone. Oily hair? Wielding any type of brush wrapped in clean gauze to absorb excess oils is more highly recommended than brushing conscientiously night and morning. Normal hair? Just continue what you've been doing; don't tamper with success. However, regardless of hair type, everyone should brush just prior to shampooing. Stimulation at that time loosens oils and buildup, facilitating cleansing.

Choose a brush according to scalp sensitivity as well as texture and length of the hair. Generally, the length of the bristles should correspond to hair length—longer hair, longer bristles. Popular club brushes, the ones usually associated with gift sets for men, are for fellows with relatively short styles. Bristle firmness should be determined by hair texture and volume. Thick, curly hair requires strong bristles; thin, fine hair needs supple bristles. For sensitive scalps, soft bristles are a must. Back to the boaring controversy: Natural bristles are very good indeed, but plastic and nylon bristles with rounded ends have been improved considerably and perform well.

Brushes, like combs, must be kept scrupulously clean. If you shampoo daily, then you should cleanse your brushes daily, too. But since you won't, at least do so once a week. Regular cleansing of brushes will help prevent the accumulation of hair strands in the bristles. These can be removed with fingers before they become plentiful. Wooden or metal handles should not be submerged in the cleansing solution. Diluted dishwater detergent or shampoo both work. Dry bristles facedown on a terry towel or upright in a glass after a complete water rinsing. Don't risk warping by placing the brush in strong artificial heat or on top of a radiator. Left to their own devices, most brushes will dry within a couple of hours.

CHAPTER 6

THE BALD TRUTH
HAIR LOSS

Even before Delilah clipped Samson, myths and theories abounded about the mysteries of hair loss. Although scientific study has progressed, determining that sex hormones contribute to characteristic male-pattern baldness in genetically predisposed men, not all factors are completely understood. Hair loss can vary among males in the same family and from generation to generation. The only foolproof—if foolhardy—solution to avoiding baldness, then, is castration prior to puberty, a drastic measure, to say the least! Some baldness is only temporary, the result of illness or trauma; growth will resume naturally. As long as the hair root (papilla) is alive, even if temporarily dormant, new growth is theoretically possible. But once the root is killed, hair revitalization is truly a dead issue.

DOWN THE DRAIN
HAIR RECESSION

Balding is not a dread disease. In fact, it's not a disease at all, although hair loss is associated with some illnesses, such as anemia and thyroid conditions (such loss is reversible by treating the disease).

Because hair pretty much grows according to an established cycle, some daily loss of hair is a healthy sign, indicating that the ongoing process of hair replenishment is taking place. Each scalp hair grows for two to six years (the average is four), then rests for about three months before being pushed out by a new hair growing from the same root. It is normal to shed between forty and sixty hairs per day, although more than this is not necessarily alarming, since over 100,000 hair follicles are found on the average head. Fortunately, follicles don't work in unison, so at any given time considerably more hairs are growing than

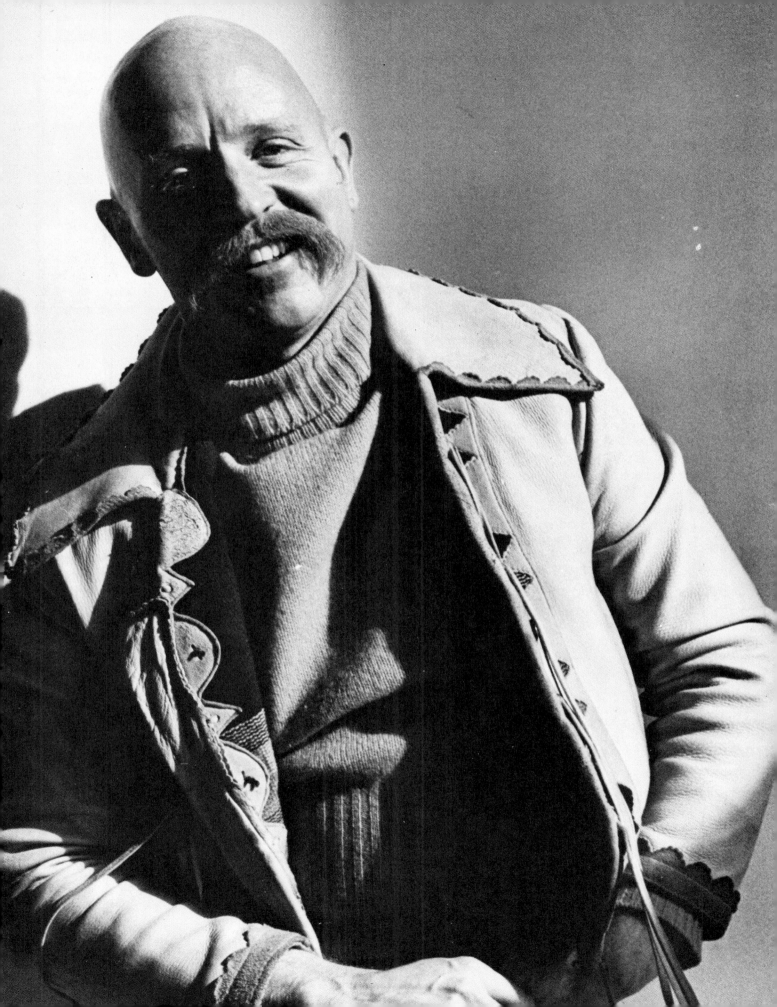

resting. However, more hairs do fall out during the autumn, perhaps a subconscious acceptance of the world's natural rhythms. Only when the rate of loss exceeds the regrowth rate does thinning or balding become evident. As men age, regrowth does slow, so thinning is inevitable.

While there are various contributory reasons for baldness, the principal one is the accumulation of androgen (the male sex hormone most related to balding) that accompanies maturation. Androgen shortens the growing phase, since the hair root is prematurely placed in the resting phase when the androgen level in the blood reaches a certain level. The more sensitive papillae—those on the crown and at the top of the forehead—are affected first, while the more hardy ones at the side of the head and at the base of the neck usually remain unperturbed. As the androgen level continues to increase, so does the frequency of resting cycles. Thus, the hair on the top of the head fails to grow to any appreciable length because the roots have atrophied, though they are not necessarily dead. The hair that is now produced looks more like fuzz than hair. Eventually this downlike growth is barely visible, although the roots keep repeating these feeble cycles of growth and rest for many years. Surprisingly, perhaps, it's very difficult to kill the papillae, and it's therefore *possible* to grow new hair on a man whose head resembles the proverbial billiard ball. If the papillae are dormant, this can be accomplished by injecting the chap with the female hormone estrogen—only he may actually start sprouting breasts, experience a reduction in his sex drive, and have other unsatisfactory side effects. Other androgen antagonists can also theoretically be injected to alleviate baldness, but there is a risk of cancer as well as femininization.

Genes also come into play in hair loss. Since the genes causing male-pattern baldness (as the name implies, most women are not affected) are inherited equally from the male and female sides, the extent of baldness and the age of its onset follow little rhyme or reason, since these genes may be recessive and thus skip one generation or one male family member, only to be dominant in another male or in another generation. Exactly how genes and androgen work together to cause baldness is largely unexplained.

When the life cycle of hair is discussed, it sounds as if the visible hair is alive too. Not so. The "life" is in the papilla, or root, which is located under the skin. It is one of the most rapidly metabolizing of the body's organs. Any change in diet or in the nervous system shows an immediate effect. That's why hair literally falls out after a severe shock. Although it cannot be definitively proved, it is likely that much hair loss is more directly attributable to stress and anxiety than it is to vitamin deficiencies, mechanical abuse, and other causes listed for premature hair loss. Charlatans, whether rogues or misguided, tend to flourish in the environment of emotionally needy guys searching for miracles.

Except for hormone shots, which have proved unacceptable, there is no actual proof that changes in the diet or mineral and vitamin supplements taken internally can alter the course of hair loss. Yet many men firmly believe in and swear by such "remedies," claiming that their hair growth has improved.

Physicians, in addition to condemning "hair vitamins" or "antibaldness lotions" as frauds, also dismiss scalp manipulation as a means to prevent or retard hair loss. Whether or not this rejection illustrates the ongoing antagonism between the scientific and cosmetics disciplines is hard to say. Physicians usually point out that the scalp has the most intricate network of blood vessels in the body, as evidenced by the gore that accompanies head wounds. Doctors simply don't accept the premise that the scalp's blood flow can be restricted and that an adequate food supply would consequently be cut off. *However*, even the most adamant detractors of scalp massage and treatments to prolong hair health do allow that these measures feel good and are relaxing. As one plastic surgeon freely admits, there is greater value in what a man perceives as truth than there is in the actual truth about baldness. Many duped men actually do find their hair growing more healthily again. Whether or not this "impossible" phenomenon is explained by the fact that the acute anxiety over hair loss has been relieved simply can't be ascertained. But some myths are absolutely unfounded. Cutting hair doesn't make it grow faster, for example, or else there'd be herds of men shaving their heads simply to cure their hair recession.

Ultimately, the question about what can and can't be done about baldness remains in the twilight zone. Scientifically, all the evidence supports the fact that, for now, there are no safe methods that are sure, despite isolated experiences suggesting otherwise. Many quacks report their cures. And so do seemingly reputable specialists. The urgency with which a man must see himself with hair will predetermine the lengths to which he'll go to try to keep or restore it. However, it should be noted that whereas most mammals need hair for warmth and protection, hair on humans is a superfluous nicety that will probably disappear eventually and entirely in future generations. Meanwhile, despite its time-honored and potent symbolism, hair or its lack proves nothing about a man's sexuality or performance abilities. If some men would worry less about hair loss, they'd likely keep more of it longer.

MAKING MORE WITH LESS

STYLING CONSIDERATIONS

With the consumer movement focusing attention on truth in packaging, perhaps it's time that some men realized that honesty in *self*-packaging can be the best policy.

Take a walk down a busy street. Look for self-packaged deceivers, guys putting on false fronts. They won't be hard to find. Odds are you'll notice men wearing ill-fitting, unkempt hairpieces or men who have nurtured the hair on one side near the back of their heads and have elaborately swirled, then plastered it forward to cover balding areas. Those men are attention grabbers, but for all the wrong reasons.

While you're looking, you'll probably also see two or three men with shining domes and voluminous muttonchop sideburns to "compensate" for top loss. They don't. They throw off the entire balance of the face and emphasize even more what's missing. Then there are the fellows with sparse, lank hair grown to near shoulder length as a strangely straggly "camouflage."

As for the men on the street wearing wigs or hairpieces or weavings or implants or transplants whom you did *not* single out as deceivers because you couldn't tell, good for them. They realize that what looks natural looks best.

There's nothing wrong with the numerous alternatives for covering up (see Chapter 7)—*if* they look natural. Unfortunately, either because of the cover-ups themselves or because of a man's failure to maintain good ones properly, many of these techniques

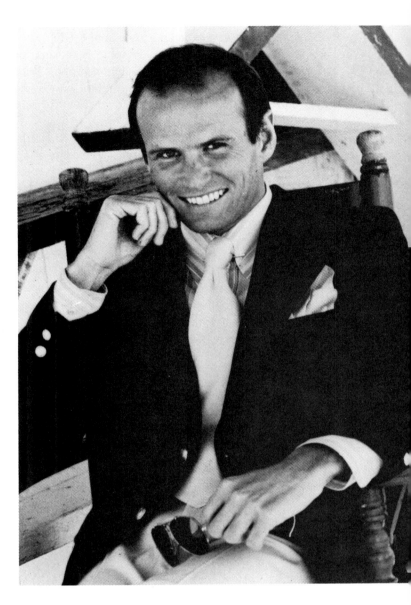

look artificial. Before going to pieces over hair loss, some might consider giving baldness a break.

Where and how balding begins will obviously indicate how the hair should be handled. In the initial stages—most men predisposed to male-pattern baldness start losing some hair as early as their teens, though not always noticeably—camouflage may indeed work well. A thinning area on the crown, for example, can usually be covered by allowing the hair to grow a little longer than normal. Or, if there's only slight recession at the temples, allowing the hair to fall easily across the forehead, then combing all the hair slightly forward, produces an attractive appearance.

Probably the worst mistake men make when hair loss graduates from mild to worrisome is teasing, or back-combing, the hair, then spraying it in place with lacquer-type products. The teasing action harms the hair, and too much spray makes even healthy hair more brittle and prone to breakage.

When hair loss becomes visibly pronounced, self-packaging dishonesty may become an obsession for some men. The classic patterns of balding—severe recession of the hairline, tending toward a horseshoe shape of balding, and/or extensive thinning on the crown in an increasingly larger circular pattern—are the ones that, without any scientific foundation, make some fellows fear the loss of their manhood. Yet, for some reason, most men feel that a thinning crown is preferable to hairline recession. Maybe because it's more visible to themselves. In either case, however, the hair is generally thinning all over the head. That's why permanents are often considered a good solution in initial and intermediary balding, for they impart body and thus give the appearance of more hair. Curls also give more coverage than does straight hair. But when the hair has atrophied and is weakened, perms are too harsh chemically and might destroy the hairs, or else the perm may simply not take. Perms can do little or nothing for severe balding.

Admittedly, on heads where hair doesn't grow, it's pointless to suggest hairstyling solutions. But in virtually every case where there's even negligible hair, a good stylist can probably achieve a positive result in place of the negatives stemming from obviously deceptive measures. Here are a couple of examples.

The Swirler

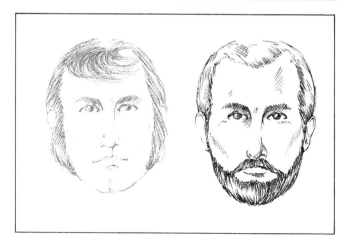

As mentioned, that ploy of camouflaging loss by training a few strands of hair to cover baldness and then adding muttonchop sideburns as compensation just doesn't work. At best, a man may look like a cartooned chipmunk. Rather than taking the defensive, a fellow might gain the offensive by treating balding as an advantage. He could have the remaining hair cut exceedingly short and forget about style all together. If the hair is dark, it can be bleached so that it doesn't look like stubble. Since the hair loss is already pronounced, the hair may already have atrophied somewhat, and bleaching may truthfully weaken it more. In this instance, however, so much the better, because the desired end is that the hair appear like downy peach fuzz. Either go with this look as it is or add a carefully groomed moustache and beard.

A Downer

When less hair is growing, it usually is a mistake to grow what's left longer, especially if the major loss is at the hairline. Since an overall thinning accompanies

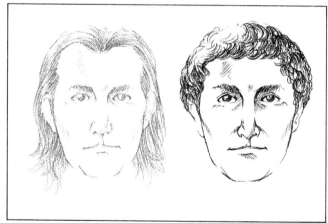

even the initial stages of baldness, when recession becomes more extensive, then longish hair on this fellow often looks stringy and unkempt, no matter what precautions are taken. Shorter hair stands up better because it automatically has more resilience and lift. It's bouncier because weighted length doesn't pull it down. Going very short, however, may present problems for the man who has pronounced features, such as enlarged ears, a jutting chin, or an oversized nose.

Off-Balance

When the hairline is receding, often it does so first at the temples, creating an exaggerated widow's peak. So how do many men try to conceal this? By combing their hair straight across the forehead from one side to the other in a very harsh line. This looks even worse if there's some wave in the hair; a viewer can begin to suffer sea sickness. Normally stylists cut hair for balance, an impossibility with unevenly receding temples. Yet the hair should be cut according to natural growth. Trying to force the hair into an unnatural shape can not only look wrong, it could prove harmful, because increased tension on the hair as it's forced into submission may cause further loss. If the hair falls naturally forward and slightly to one side, the most pleasing method of capitalizing on the hair recession is to emphasize the face asymmetrically by keeping the temple high on one side and combing the hair across to the other side, avoiding a well-defined hairline. Allowing one area to appear thinner than the other will make a man look less bald, not more so.

Crowned

If hair loss is so advanced that major "camouflage" is required, forget about it, for trying to pass off a small amount of hair for a headful is a fool's mission. However, the hair can be cut to redirect the eye from the baldness to another area of the head. Certainly this is true with a balding crown. Conjure up an image of Norse Vikings. The image is invariably virile, and the first thought is of rather full hair covering part of the ears and turning inward to frame the face. That baldness at the crown comes second or third in the recollection. The absolute reverse impression comes

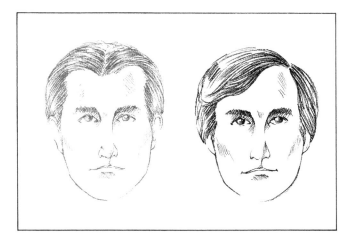

from a conservative, dull style combed back from the face in a vain attempt to make a bald crown appear less vulnerable. It only looks sadder. Of course, wearing a Viking-type style can be too extreme for a short, frail man, but he can adapt the idea by keeping the hair neatly clipped (remember, the shorter the style, the more bounce to the hair, hence the impression of more hair) with some extra fullness at the sides so that the hair grazes the ears. If the temples are likewise more bare than hairy, he might try the asymmetrical trick with a side part. This will help create a new facial focus, leading the eye to what hair he has rather than to where he hasn't any.

Vanishing Act

There's yet another way to beat baldness without going to pieces. Welcome it. Especially young men who've experienced premature hair loss might consider shaving it *all* off. Then baldness doesn't appear to be an untimely fluke. Instead, it expresses strong-willed determination and a forceful personality.

CHAPTER 7
UNDERCOVER AGENTS
HAIR REPLACEMENT

There's no such thing as a good cover-up if someone can detect it. Yet many men would rather risk discovery than face the ridicule of baldness. Whether sneers and sniggers would necessarily materialize is incidental: These fellows can't bear to grin and bare it. If someone is psychologically ill equipped to handle balding, he should investigate the various cover-ups immediately once it's clear that the thinning is irreversible. Putting hair back on a very bald head is far more shocking than taking early corrective steps. Choosing the right technique from the several available isn't easy, since each alternative by its own nature has inherent pros and cons.

OVERALLS
WIGS

Unlike toupees, which are principally designed to cover a man's balding area, wigs are created to cover the entire hair zone from the forehead to the back of the neck. Most are on stretch caps, and recently some makers have incorporated "skin" portions from the hairline to the crown. (*Skin* is an industry term referring to a thin membrane of lightly tinted urethane through which replacement hair is sewn; when worn, the true scalp skin shows through, giving a natural appearance.) In the past, many men's wigs were simply cut-down versions of women's. The results weren't very appealing. But technological improvements have been made.

In the forefront of many men's-wig innovations has been a young team, Ron Barris and John Zervoulei, co-partners of Headstart Hair for Men, which produces and distributes handmade wigs and hairpieces sold around the country in hair salons. The two also operate a retail establishment, Barris & Zervoulei Hair for Men, in New York City.

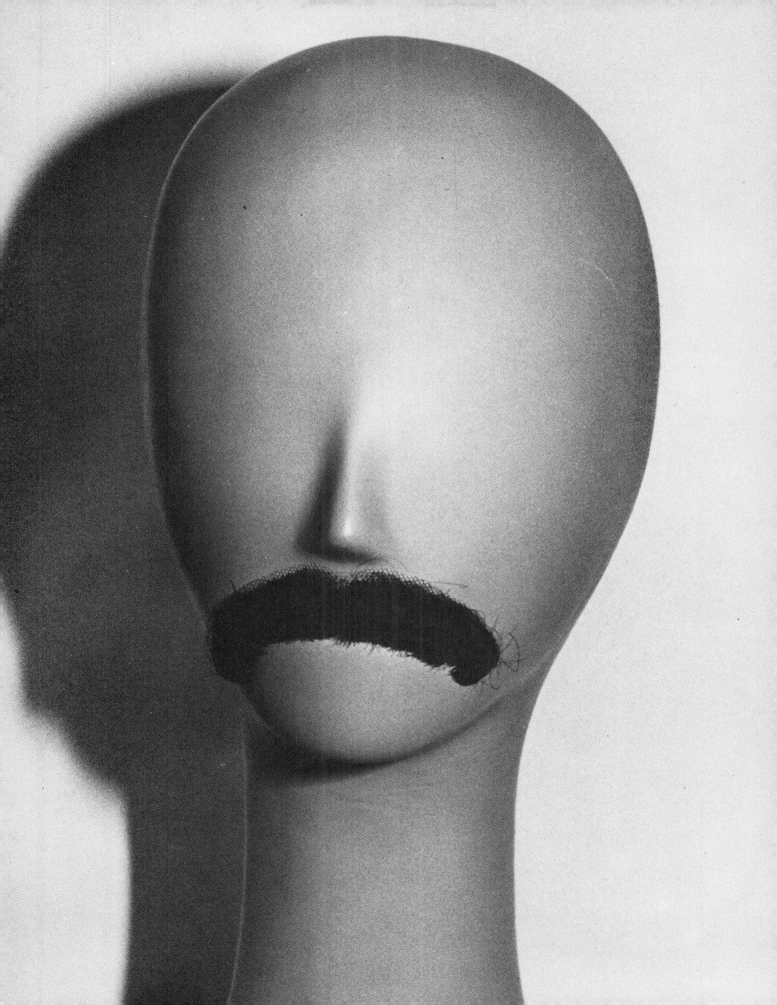

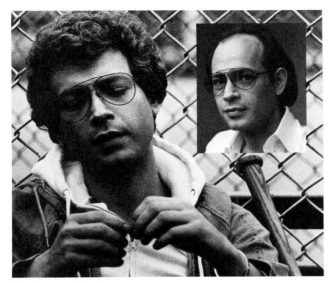

© 1977 by Bill Cahill

John explains that male wig purchasers, whether very bald or simply receding, "want an 'unachievable' look they could never have gotten from their real hair. It's a stylized look. Men who buy wigs don't want a short, conservative IBM style. Nor is that desirable, since it doesn't take advantage of what wigs offer— lots of versatility because of the hair length. It's true that wigs can be cut quite short, but that rather defeats one of their reasons for being."

Mentioning that Headstart Hair's two most popular wig models are the Combo (a stretch wig able to be combed in any direction, so the hair can be center-, left-, or right-parted, or brushed back without a part) and the Curly (which, as its name implies, is a precurled, carefree style), John says both are handmade on stretch bases with transparent "skin" tops. He strongly endorses synthetic modacrylic fibers for wigs, claiming that they are easier to care for and more versatile.

"Strangely, synthetic fibers imitate human hair far better than human hair does," John insists. "With human hair wigs or hairpieces, to get the necessary coverage, makers must use more hair than with synthetics. The result is a denser-looking wig or piece that just doesn't look natural. Besides, human hair fades more quickly than synthetics. Some people say there's an unnatural luster to synthetics, but this need not be. Proper blending of the shades is what counts. You'd never want a wig in a single hair shade, because real hair has many different tones in it. One mistake many men make when buying a wig or any other replace-

ment is that they want the hair color they had before. It's usually too dark. As men age, some pigment is lost. Their skins also become more sallow. A color one or two shades lighter than what they had in their teens always looks better. A lighter shade also counterbalances any 'wigginess' that a deep, dark, dense mass of hair can give even if the hair is a man's own."

Wigs are unquestionably the easiest hair replacements to buy. The procedure is usually as follows.

1

A man simply decides he's interested in a wig, then visits several local outlets to compare their wares. Even though some fine pieces are sold via direct-mail advertising, it is still advisable to check out wigs in person.

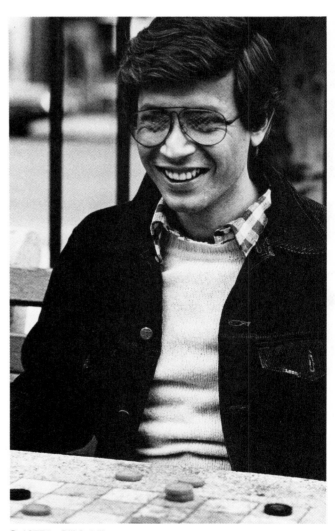

© 1977 by Bill Cahill

2

A man should try on several styles and shades until he's grown accustomed to his face with hair again. At first the impression may be one of drastic change, so he should take his time and study his appearance. A salesman should show him how to position the wig correctly, since most men will put it too far down on the forehead. If a fellow has his own hairline, he should experiment with brushing some of that hair into the wig. Is the blending successful? Do the sideburns color-match?

3

Unhappy? Leave. Or try on a different wig. Or consider a different technique. Happy? Buy it. But not before learning how to manipulate the wig and how to take care of it.

Pros & Cons

"A man must become involved to receive maximum satisfaction from a wig or any other kind of hair replacement," suggests John. "Primarily that includes caring for it himself. Wigs should be brushed every morning and evening to keep the hair loose. And they should be cleaned once or twice a week. Shampooing in the sink with a mild liquid dishwashing detergent, conditioning with a diluted fabric softener, rinsing thoroughly, and then draping the wig over a bottle for air drying are all very easy steps. Blow drying is not recommended, since the heat may straighten the wig's hair. Men should never sleep in wigs, which flattens and mats them."

Since most wigs are worn daily, they should be replaced every year or so. It is also advisable for a wig wearer to return every two or three months to the shop where it was purchased so the piece can be examined for any fiber loss or for reshaping. If any recurling or rewaving is needed, this can be done at the salon. Men can also do this themselves with a Teflon-coated curling iron, but they must be especially careful. If the heat setting is too high, the fibers may be scorched or otherwise destroyed.

Because of their stretch bases, wigs feel rather secure on the head but may not be. Wigs with "skin" grip better because of the texture of the urethane against the scalp. Nonetheless, for extra security some men resort to toupee tape to further fasten a wig. But tape attached to the scalp over existing hair can accelerate hair loss through pulling and tearing. Clips are slightly less dangerous, although they too can place too much strain on existing hair. Some wigs come with small barrette combs as anchors to eliminate the tendency of the piece to ride up the back of the head. Since hair in this area is generally not subject to male-pattern baldness, there is little potential for harm.

Although "skin" wigs look more natural, they are also more fragile. Hair loss from the wigs themselves is faster: The hair fibers cannot be double-knotted since they would be too bulky and might destroy the smooth "scalp" appearance.

Wigs are definitely warmer to wear than hairpieces, so there is a greater hazard of discomfort. On the other hand, wigs are more easily removed than hairpieces, so there should be no odor problem if the scalp is cleansed regularly on a day-to-day basis.

Wig wearers should not wear caps or hats. These increase perspiration and flatten the style. Unsecured wigs might also be accidentally removed with the hat or the cap.

PIECE & HAPPINESS
HAIRPIECES

While wigs are created to cover a man's entire hair area, with hairpieces the replacement hair blends into some of the fellow's existing growth. Formerly called toupees and still occasionally derogatorily referred to as rugs, hairpieces come in different sizes and types. A full piece (primarily designed to disguise horseshoe baldness) creates a hairline, covers the crown, and blends into the sideburns and the hair at the base of the skull. A partial piece conceals isolated baldness, say at the crown, or supplements thinning hair to add fullness and to hide the emerging scalp. Oversized pieces fit atop nearly three-quarters of the head or more, even though baldness may not be that advanced. The piece's base can vary from delicate silk and lace for custom-made versions to nylon mesh for ready-made models.

Custom-made hairpieces are currently on the decline because of the expense, their relative fragility,

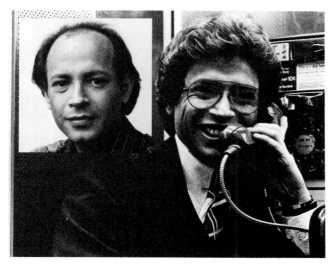

© 1977 by Bill Cahill

and the inroads being made by improved ready-made ones. Nonetheless, some men insist that hairpieces require as much individual fitting as do dentures and eyeglasses. Such fellows still follow the custom route. The procedure, as done at Barris & Zervoulei Hair for Men, follows.

1

The patron is seated in a barber's chair while the operator, using a square of clear plastic wrap, stretches this material over the bald area, pulling the wrap and ridding it of any wrinkles until it is smooth and formfitting. This ensures that the base of the hairpiece will correspond to the patron's head shape and original hairline.

2

Now tape is used to duplicate the configuration of the patron's head. Beginning at the forehead, tape is placed on the wrap over what will become the outer perimeters of the final piece. These boundaries are determined by the extent of baldness.

3

Next the inner portion of the wrap is completely covered with overlapping strips of tape, turning the wrap into a transparent, three-dimensional mold of the patron's balding zone.

4

The mold is placed on the patron's head again. The operator traces with a felt-tip pen the dimensions of the baldness. He also delineates where the front hairline should begin (generally four fingers above the brow line), draws an appropriate part line, and indicates the client's original growth pattern on the crown.

5

The completed mold is removed and trimmed. At this point there are various alternatives. The pattern can be measured against a standard, ready-made hairpiece so that the piece can be trimmed into a semi-custom one. Or a completely custom hairpiece can be designed.

6

If the client opts for a completely custom-made piece, the contoured mold of the man's bald area is traced onto a wooden form. Such wood blocks look somewhat like featureless mannequins. The foundation material, whether nylon net, gauze, lace, silk, or urethane, is attached to the mold. Ribbon or half binding is usually added around the edges of the foundation for dimensional stability, and the base is then sewn by hand.

7

At this point the piece is ready for hair to be inserted. The process of sewing in hair is called ventilation, actually a hand-crocheting action. (The hair, whether synthetic or human, has been previously color-matched. This blending is crucial to a natural appearance.)

8

After the hair has been inserted—usually it is eight to ten inches long for handling ease—there is some prestyling, cutting the hair to the client's specification, but most often leaving it about one-half to one inch longer than expected wearing length so that the final styling can be done atop the client's head.

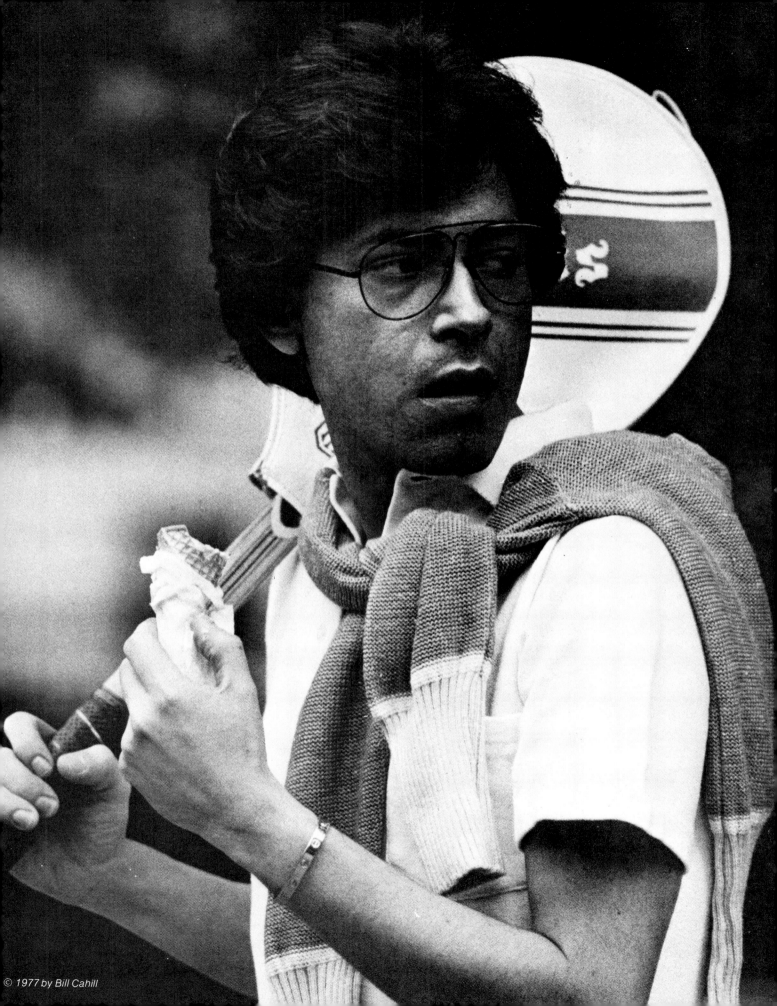

9

When the hairpiece is completed, the customer returns to the salon for the final styling. (If the piece had been trimmed from a ready-made type, this step would directly follow step 5.) First the piece is properly positioned on his head. Two-way transparent tape, applied in two strips at the front of the piece and one in the back, attach the hairpiece to the scalp. Before the hairpiece is positioned, however, an alcohol-saturated cotton ball removes excess oil from the scalp.

10

Correctly in place, the piece is now fully styled on the patron's head, with special care given to feathering the piece to blend with the client's natural hair.

Any hairpiece demands care and maintenance, and those custom-made with fragile silk or lace bases require even more. When removed, the tape should also be taken off, otherwise a sticky buildup results. Most makers caution against shampooing human-hair pieces, and this means more return visits to the salon for upkeep. Hair loss is inevitable, so these pieces must also periodically be returned to the salon for additional hair and even dyeing to counteract oxidation. Thus many men need two hairpieces in order to have one to wear while the other is being cleaned or repaired. The lifespan of a hairpiece is difficult to gauge. Three years is absolutely the maximum, with one year perhaps optimum for having the piece look its best.

For these sundry reasons, the aforementioned hair replacement innovators, Barris & Zervoulei, are increasingly spending their energies in improving ready-made hairpieces. They claim that such hand-made pieces can retain quality craftsmanship while being more accessible to clients' desires and wallets. Their part-anywhere hairpiece is just that. It can be cut down for a semicustomized fit; and the rather longish style can be trimmed to a very conservative look. With a lightweight urethane skin base from hairline to crown, it—like the Headstart Hair for Men wigs—is made in many shades of synthetic mod-acrylic fiber.

"Younger men have fewer problems with psycho-logical adjustments to wearing pieces," notes Ron Barris. "Older men tend to wear their hairpieces constantly, which is bad, because nothing looks worse than a hairpiece that isn't taken care of."

Pros & Cons

Custom-made pieces of human hair are far more difficult to maintain than the ready-made synthetics. For either, proper care and proper fit go hand in hand as the keys to success.

Like wigs, hairpieces should be brushed night and morning. If synthetic, they should be shampooed once or twice weekly. Human-hair pieces can be cleaned by immersion in a dry-cleaning solution. However, restyling is then necessitated, and many men simply can't cope.

Despite cartoons depicting embarrassed men chasing their toupees down the street, a hairpiece nearly always holds firmly in place except during sports or physical exertion (and that may include *that*): Perspiration can dislodge the tape and cause the piece to slip.

The most common mistake by wearers—other than failing to take adequate care of the piece—is placing it too far down on the forehead, the "sin of the absent forehead," notes Ron. "The maxim for correct placement is three fingers from the eyebrows to the fringe of hair, four fingers to the base."

Initially a man should expect to spend a minimum of ten minutes positioning a hairpiece, but eventually placement will become second nature, almost like putting on a hat. Of course, mirrors are mandatory to confirm the verdict.

The giveaway faults with hairpieces are the hard line at the hairline and the crucial part line. Properly constructed and fitting pieces should not have these drawbacks.

The prime advantages of hairpieces over wigs are their more comfortable, lighter weight and their adaptability to more conservative styling. Since hairpieces are easily removed, the scalp can be properly cleansed. Special care should be given to removing all traces of tape by using cotton balls soaked in an alcohol-based liquid. Hairpieces, like wigs, should not be worn to bed. Nor should hair spray be used to keep them in place, since the piece may then look dull and artificial.

TOGETHERNESS
HAIRWEAVING

Hairweaving is another nonsurgical solution for covering baldness by literally weaving replacement hair onto the perimeter of a man's own existing hair. Several variations exist in the technique. An older method, called line-by-line weaving, involves braiding an "edge" of hair surrounding the balding area; then wefts of replacement hair (individual hairs attached to a strip) are attached to this edge in a side-by-side manner. The result is a rather flat style requiring hair spray to keep it in place.

A more advanced procedure, as performed at The Hair Club for Men Ltd. in New York City, is named the strand-by-strand weaving method.

"Strand-by-strand hairweaving is for any balding or bald man, but particularly for younger guys who, like myself, have experienced hair loss in their twenties and just aren't psychologically suited to hairpieces," relates Sy Sperling, president of the firm. "These men need to feel that the hair is their own, not something they can take on and off like a hat. Admittedly, hairweaving is more complicated than wearing a hairpiece, but the results are more natural and the feeling is more secure."

The first steps in hairweaving, however, are much the same as when ordering a custom-made hairpiece.

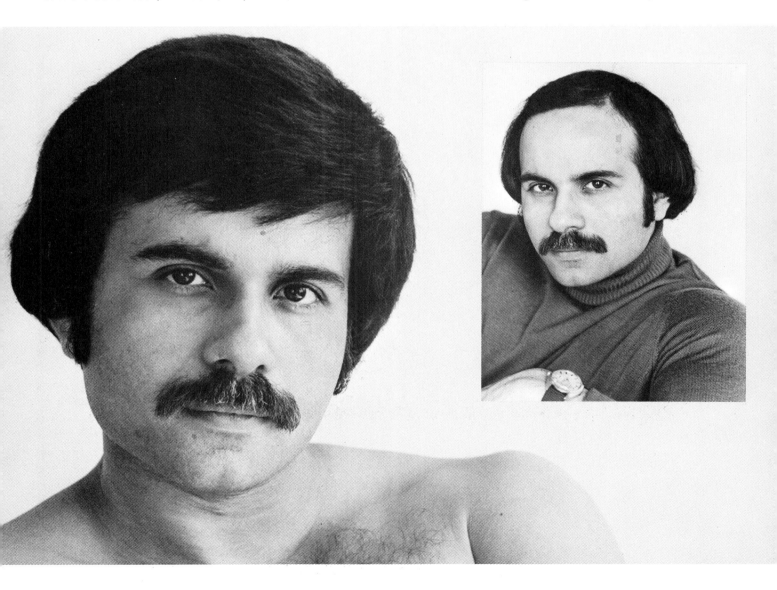

1

After deciding upon this form of hair replacement, the client makes an appointment with an established firm for measurements. Using clear plastic wrap and tape, the practitioner makes a contoured mold of the balding area and marks the mold with a felt-tip pen to note details about the perimeter of the baldness and the natural hair growth.

2

At the same time small snippets of hair are cut from various parts of the head. These will be used to ensure the closest possible color blend between replacement and natural hair.

3

The client leaves, but work continues. Using the mold as a pattern, a porous webbing of filaments is cut precisely to the dimension of the man's baldness.

4

Following natural growth direction, the custom-blended replacement hair is handwoven strand by strand into the webbing.

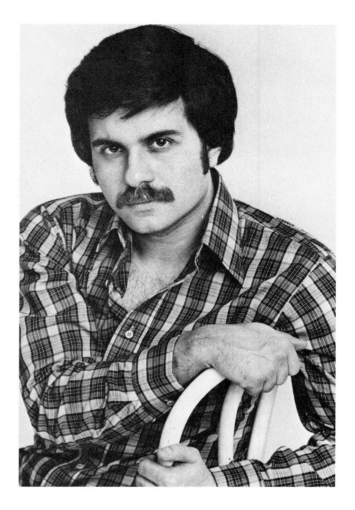

5

When the client returns, the replacement piece is ready, although its hair has been left longer than expected wearing length so that styling can be finalized atop the man's head. However, first the technician braids a powerful-but-thin nylon thread into the hair around the balding area, creating a continuous "edge." The goal is to keep this braid as flat and as close to the scalp as possible.

6

Now the replacement process is attached by interweaving it with the woven braid of nylon and hair. (Strictly speaking, because the weave is neither a wig nor a hairpiece, it is termed a replacement process.) This step is also done gently by hand. Great care must be taken to secure the process with enough tautness to make it feel snug without being painful and without placing too much tension on the surrounding natural hair.

7

Conforming closely and firmly to the scalp's contours, the replacement is now ready for final styling to the man's features and personality.

"There are several misconceptions about hairweaving," says Sy. "Some people believe that hairweaving accelerates further hair loss due to increased tension on the existing hair, causing it to weaken and eventually break. That happens only if the operator is inexperienced. The process should only be woven into existing strong hair, not at the forehead or temples. Tape will secure it at the hairline. And since the natural hair is growing, some of the tension will automatically lessen, though the weave won't slip or slide."

Pros & Cons

A reported disadvantage in hairweaving is that repeated returns to the shop are required to keep the weave in shape. To some extent, this is very true, since the natural hair continues growing, thereby loosening the process and necessitating retightening, which a man can't perform himself. Maintenance therefore does increase the initial cost.

"Yet, depending on the man, these return visits average from between six to eight or ten weeks," counters Sy. "Nonbalding men probably go to a barber at least that frequently. Besides, the growing natural hair has to be trimmed, which can be done at the same time the weave is being tightened."

Improper cleansing of the scalp—and washing beneath the weave takes patience, agility, and thoroughness—potentially leads to bacteria buildup, irritation, and an unpleasant odor. Does Sy deny this? "Not at all," he answers, "but the incidence is rare. And that's the fault of the man, not the process. The drawback of *all* hair replacements is abuse by the wearer. Reputable establishments educate their clients and insist that they take all the proper precautions."

Hairweavings can—and *must*—be shampooed regularly at home to maintain natural luster and movement. Mild shampoos should be used, since the naturally secreted oils from the scalp don't offer as much protection to replacement hair. Fingers must push beneath the weave to massage the shampoo onto the scalp. Jet action water sprays make the mandatory thorough rinsing easier. An instant conditioner is also highly recommended after each shampoo to untangle the hair, add luster, and make the weave more manageable. Lacquertype hair sprays are too abrasive for replacement hair, although some lanolin-finish sprays will help hold the hair in place while protecting it from sunlight and oxidation. Combs, especially metal ones without any give, shouldn't be used, since their teeth may catch in the webbing and yank the weave, breaking the replacement hair and pulling the wearer's own. Blow dryers are acceptable if the replacement hair is of the human variety, and if the implements are held at a safe distance—about ten inches to a foot away. Unlike the recommended method for using a blow dryer on natural hair, the prescribed technique for a man with a weave is to direct the nozzle directly toward the scalp (but at a lower setting than usual) in order to remove the excess moisture and ensure drying from the scalp out. Styling should also be done at reduced settings for greater control.

The most successful style for a hairweave is ear grazing so that the replacement hair can casually blend with the man's sideburns and existing hair. This minimizes any textural variation that may occur due to humidity or perspiration, when the natural hair responds to nature but the replacement hair doesn't. (This potential problem is inherent in any hair replacement if the style is too short and consequently the added hair can't form a "union" with the real hair.) Since the replacement process moves away from the scalp and needs retightening as the natural hair grows, this is another reason why trying for too conservative or closely cropped a hairstyle seldom works.

The most successful style for a hairweave is ear grazing so that the replacement hair can casually blend with the man's sideburns and existing hair. This minimizes any textural variation that may occur due to humidity or perspiration, when the natural hair responds to nature but the replacement hair doesn't. (This potential problem is inherent in any hair replacement if the style is too short and consequently the added hair can't form a "union" with the real hair.) Since the replacement process moves away from the scalp and needs retightening as the natural hair grows, this is another reason why trying for too conservative or closely cropped a hairstyle seldom works.

"Men shouldn't expect miracles from hairweaves or any hair replacement," advises Sy. "For the man who's willing to expend no energy, the results will be close to zero, whatever alternative he chooses to cover his baldness. But for the guy who's committed to looking good, which means caring for his hairweave, the results of this procedure in skilled hands can be excellent. Some people say human hair is more difficult to care for than synthetic. Perhaps so. But quality human hair used for hairweaving looks and feels more natural to the touch; can be better matched in texture and color to a man's own hair simply because it's human hair, after all; reacts better to hair conditioners; and performs better in the wind. We've experimented with synthetic hair and don't like the results. It might be easier, but easier doesn't mean better."

A STITCH IN TIME
HAIR IMPLANTATION

Hair implantation has been described as the least desirable approach to covering baldness. Harsh words, and not necessarily true. The success of implants, a quasi-surgical technique, depends on where the procedure is performed and under what conditions. By its nature, implantation involves *potential* difficulties that may or may not materialize, depending upon the professionalism and expertise of the practitioner. (Since implantation should be performed by a physician, no particular implantation center will be named.)

Unfortunately, because of the similarity in the names, implantation is often confused with transplantation. Transplantation is a totally surgical method that literally involves relocating growing hair from donor sites to nongrowing areas. Implantation is minor cosmetic surgery to affix matching hair to the scalp. Strips of hair (called wefts) are anchored by "retainers," surgical threads implanted in the scalp tissues surrounding the balding area. The procedure is as follows.

1

A man considering hair implantation makes an appointment for a consultation. He is under no obligation, and no fee should be involved. The entire procedure is explained. The man should request to see "before and after" photographs of individuals who have undergone the procedure. The potential client's medical history is (or should be) explored to ascertain if any recurrent health problems would dictate against the process. If the man has any serious scalp disorder, he is (or should be) dissuaded from implantation until the condition is alleviated.

2

Should the man choose to undergo implantation, he describes the type of hairstyle he wants, since the pattern of the implantation affects the visual outcome. Usually a hair stylist is present to offer assistance.

3

A transparent mold of his bald area is taken in a similar manner to the initial stages of custom hair-pieces or hairweaving. This contoured measurement will be marked to indicate where the anchors should be positioned in his scalp. These anchors, or retainers, are also often called sutures (which is different from the medical term that refers to the strands used for sewing up a wound).

4

Small snippets are cut from the man's hair so that the replacement hair can be carefully blended to match his natural color. Often several shades from the same color family must be blended to achieve the desired results.

5

The man schedules an appointment for the minor surgery. It should be performed only by a qualified physician. Most professional implantation centers have arrangements with one or several doctors, who do the medical part of the implanting. This is often executed at the center, not in the physician's office.

6

After the client leaves, trained technicians create handwoven strips of the specially blended hair. These wefts will be affixed to retainers following surgery.

7

Returning to the implantation center, the man is taken to a private room, where he meets the physician. (The client has every right to ask to see the doctor's professional resume prior to this stage.) A nurse should be in attendance. A local anesthetic is injected into the scalp. Some discomfort is not uncommon.

8

When the scalp is totally anesthetized, the surgical threads are placed in the scalp around the balding area and strategically within it. The pattern is generally circular. Although initially wires were employed, today the threadlike retainers are more flexible and lie closer to the surface of the scalp.

9

The wefts of blended hair are now attached to the retainers.

After the procedure is completed, the client is allowed to rest before being taken to the styling room, where the replacement hair is cut and shaped with his natural hair.

Under optimum conditions, the resulting implant will remain in place and perform satisfactorily for several years.

Under the worst conditions, however, an immediate infection may ensue. *Or* the man may not be able to tolerate the weight of the wefts. *Or* the retainers may break. *Or* any number of horror tales. But just because these unfortunate events have been known to occur doesn't mean they necessarily will. Nevertheless, when considering implantation, a man must be doubly convinced that the center performing the service is reputable and experienced.

Pros & Cons

The most appealing aspect of hair implantation is that the replacement hair is more "permanent" than that acquired with wigs, pieces, or hairweaving. Not to be taken on and off, an implant *can't* be removed daily or weekly. The implant will not loosen with natural hair growth, although pulling on the retainers with shampooing and brushing *may* eventually weaken them, possibly causing some breakage. New retainers must then be implanted, although the broken ones must first be removed.

Cleansing is not especially easy but no more time-consuming or difficult than with a hairweave. In fact, since with implantation no webbing covers the scalp, gently massaging the shampoo under the wefts might be a little easier. However, lifting the wefts must be done gently. Straining the anchors is inadvisable and can be painful, like yanking your own hair.

Most implantation currently involves the use of synthetic hair since it is less affected by oxidation. Shampooing frequency depends upon the condition of the natural hair. However, blow drying is very dangerous for synthetic hair. Curling irons are verboten. The most thorough drying technique is first to blot the hair gently with a terry towel, then to blot it again, weft by weft, with an absorbent paper towel. Combing isn't recommended, since the teeth may catch in the wefts. Small, specially designed natural-bristle brushes style implants nicely.

The versatility of styles achievable through implantation is not as extensive as with wigs or hairpieces.

Since the physician supervising the retainer implants will try to keep their number at a minimum, this necessitates relatively longer hair strands so that no "spotty" areas are visible, which would mean exposure of the scalp and/or the retainers. Very short, conservative styles won't work. If the baldness covers most of the crown, no true part is possible. If the baldness encompasses the hairline, off-the-face styles must be tousled.

Like any replacement and even some human hair, implants tend to mat during a night's sleep. They should be brushed regularly and "finger-styled" throughout the day.

Implants have worked successfully for a number of men. However, certain fellows with tender scalps have found the technique painful. Guys who enjoy active sports are warned to resist the temptation to implant, since rough treatment on the retainers never provokes laughter. In addition, heavy perspiration will change the texture of natural hair but not that of the implant, making the replacement particularly self-advertising.

Should a man be unhappy with the results of an implant, the retainers can be removed, but usually there will be scarring.

SUPPLY AND DEMAND
HAIR TRANSPLANTATION

Transplantation rightly sounds a bit like gardening. Just as healthy plants can be uprooted from one plot and transferred to new soil, a man's thriving hair is taken from one fertile area of the head (usually from the base of the back neck) and rooted anew on his balding area. A surgical treatment for male-pattern baldness, hair transplantation should only be performed by a qualified dermatologist, physician, or plastic surgeon.

Notice the way that very bald men, whose crowns are totally devoid of any visible growth, almost always have fairly dense fringes of hair at the sideburns, around the ears, and at the back of the neck. Inexplicably, these fringes are unaffected by common male-pattern baldness. Since hair growth is programmed in the hair root, transplanted hair from the "fringe" remains programmed to grow wherever relocated, provided the root survives the move intact.

Since genetic receptivity must be ensured, hair can only be transplanted onto the same head, not from one man to another. One exception: A possible donor could be an identical twin, but brotherly love has its limits.

Although a relatively expensive procedure (usually calculated on a per-plug basis), hair transplantation is today the most common cosmetic operation for men. A detailed step-by-step description of the procedure, however, might cause the technique to become the least sought baldness alternative. The scalp is abundantly blessed with blood vessels, so the procedure is quite gory and not for the queasy. Nor is it for the impatient.

Since it is impracticable to transplant individual hairs follicle by follicle, small pieces of the scalp containing a number of hair follicles are removed from the donor site with a cylindrical punch that's about $\frac{5}{32}$ inch in diameter. The same punch has already been used to bore out a specified number of plugs of bald scalp in the receptor area, into which the grafts are relocated. (More precisely stated, hair transplants are really scalp transplants.) Theoretically, it's possible to transplant up to 150 grafts per session, although during the first session far fewer will probably be transplanted. Some physicians prefer doing only thirty or so.

As stated, the process is bloody. But the gore has its value, since some practitioners allow the congealing blood to secure the grafts in place. Others may suture the sites; such sutures are later removed and do not affect the hair growth.

Following the session, nonsticky dressings are placed over the donor and receptor areas. Some doctors recommend removing all bandages and dressings the morning after the transplantation. Others suggest keeping the head swaddled for a week. Either way, care must be taken not to disturb the grafts, which are now encrusted with dried blood—not an especially appetizing sight. When these scabs eventually fall off—usually after a week or two—secure attachment of the plugs has taken place. However, if our patient hasn't listened carefully to the transplantation scenario, he's in for a shock. All the transplanted hair stubs fall out within a few weeks to two months after surgery. This phenomenon doesn't signify a horrendous failure but is part of the normal course of events. The trauma of transplantation forces the hair root into a dormant stage. The old hair works its way out of the pore. But a healthy root will commence growing a new hair shaft shortly. Still, it may be up to a year before the full effects of transplantation are visible.

Unfortunately, not all hair roots survive the trip. Each plug contains between twelve and eighteen roots. Between six and fourteen of them usually sprout, although some patients average as little as three to four hairs per plug. On the other hand, up to fifteen or sixteen growing roots per plug have been reported. Chances of no growth whatsoever are infinitesimal if the practitioner is experienced.

Transplanted hair is as hale and hearty as normal hair, simply because that's precisely what it is. It can be colored, permed, what-have-you-ed, with no more nor less risk than untransplanted hair. Since the transplanted root, if intact, is not affected by male-pattern baldness, the hair should grow permanently. However, other hair may not. As male-pattern baldness progresses at its predetermined rate, additional hair loss will probably ensue. Starting transplantation sessions early in the balding process means that fewer graftings will be needed per session, thereby extending expense and discomfort gradually over an extended period of time. Of course, the potential source of supply diminishes with each and every graft, since hair roots are only rearranged and not numerically increased.

All transplant practitioners have their own techniques. Some work in tandem with hair stylists from the outset. Others rely on their own judgment and experience in placing the plugs. Creating a straight hairline and ignoring the rest of the head shows poor planning. The art of the technique is as important as the medical expertise. A prospective patient should always ask to be shown 'before and after' photographs of men who have undergone the procedure under the particular doctor's hands. Never should transplantation be entrusted to someone without the proper credentials.

Pros & Cons

Transplantation is the only baldness remedy that utilizes a man's own hair as the sole solution. Since the transplanted hair is growing and real, no special maintenance is required other than a sensible hair care regimen.

Transplants are not cheap. However, the initial cost

increases only when further grafts are necessary. Thus, the expense is amortized over a lifetime.

Men with pronounced horseshoe baldness should recognize that their hair loss may be so advanced that transplantation can only result in skimpy hair coverage. It's far wiser to forego the procedure entirely than to start it and then stop midway. Periodic, widely spaced tufts of hair look worse than no hair at all.

Since the hair texture from the donating fringe is often coarser than hair atop the head, the transplanted hair may be a bit harder to manage than the hair that used to top the head.

Some men have found the process painful. Success cannot be guaranteed. However, after suffering through the initial discomfort (patients shouldn't bend or strain excessively for about a week following each grafting session), most men have been quite satisfied with transplants. Remember, transplantation is surgery. Its results can only be as safe as the doctor performing it is competent.

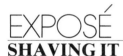

EXPOSÉ
SHAVING IT

Baldness is not a heinous crime. Some men look terrific bald. Some men don't look terrific even with hair.

Bad coverups are baldly offensive. How does someone know how he'll look *totally* bald until he's tried it? Shaving the head doesn't destroy the hair roots or program the hair any differently. Trimming off the fringes with scissors, then shaving the head with an electric razor is the ultimate exposé. Of course, head shaving should be performed daily to avoid cranial five o'clock shadow. The fringe will always grow back if the results of head shaving are unappealing. Then, the guy must either accept fate or try for a fateful change with one of the several cover-up methods discussed.

Pros & Cons

If the skull's shape is abnormal, head shaving accentuates the unfortunate configuration. But if the shape is from acceptable to great, the results of head shaving might be acceptable to great. Shaving the head every day isn't fun, but going through the motions with hair replacements isn't loads of yuks either.

Regardless of what a man does about his baldness, he should not allow the countermeasures to become obsessions. He should periodically remind himself that balding does *not* banish him to a life of shame and ridicule. Jeers only erupt when someone appears vulnerable—and foolish—by going to foppish extremes. Self-confidence is a tremendous asset in looking good. It's also the best defense against cranks: *They* are the jerks, not the bald ones. Anyway, their noses look like pickles.

CHAPTER 8

FRINGE BENEFITS
FACIAL HAIR

At a distant point in prehistory, some foolish fellows started yanking the hairs from their faces with clamshells. *Voilà*, the visible face came into fashion. Although modern shaving is far easier than the weird methods practiced in antiquity, some residual primitive instinct still causes beards and moustaches to grow back into popularity from time to time. Today facial hair is a question of whatever makes your boat float.

HOME GROWN
BEARDS & MOUSTACHES

When first growing a beard or a moustache, a man should be prepared for this hair to be a different shade than the hair atop his head. Seldom, if ever, do the two match.

Nor should someone expect the same set of problems for both skull and facial hair. On the plus side, beards are seldom inclined toward excessive oiliness. However, the face is much more tender than the scalp. Beard coarseness can be irritating; if the whiskers are curly, ingrown hairs can blight the benefits of adding fringe.

The way to grow a beard or moustache is simply to stop shaving the areas of desired growth. For those interested in moustaches only, the smile lines generally form the outer perimeters of where not to shave. Beard fanciers shouldn't shave at all for three or four weeks. Some men try shaping facial hair immediately. A waste of time, since ingrowing hair looks scrubby no matter what. Some density is necessary before styling. Beard growth varies from man to man, yet expecting decent results in less than six weeks is unrealistic. Patience, pal.

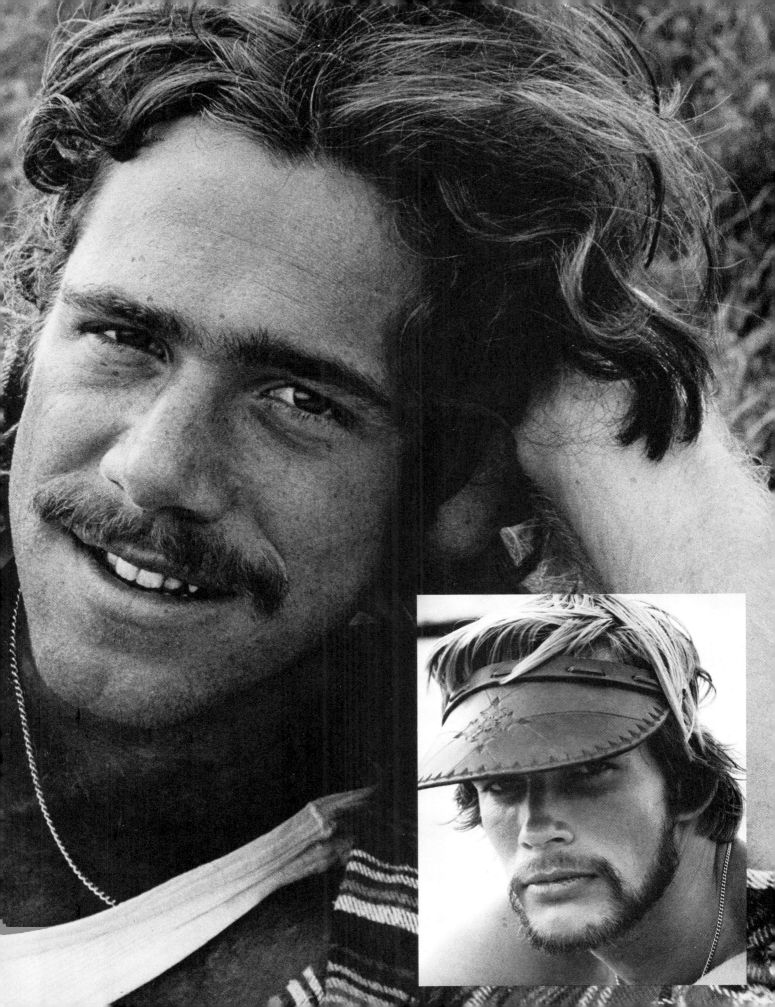

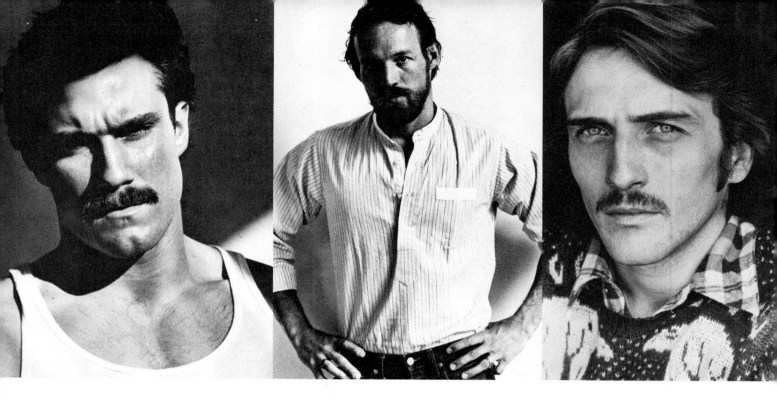

After stubble advances past prickles and blooms into an approximation of full whiskers, then a fellow can start calculating the image he wants to present. The choices are wide, though some are wide of the mark any guy should want to make.

One out-of-date moustache style is the familiar very short, straight growth on the upper lip. When exceedingly thin, it resembles the type worn by Clark Gable during the late thirties, a look immortalized on "The Late Show." With a bit more depth, it recalls Charlie Chaplin's "Little Tramp."

Its opposite style is the walrus moustache. Big and brash, it seldom looks trimmed and usually isn't. On a small man, it looks ridiculous. It can on larger men, too. Not an easy style to carry off, a walrus moustache invariably looks as if it belongs to a character actor.

Handlebar moustaches are walruses tamed, usually with wax to shape them. Unless someone sings in a barbershop quartet regularly, handlebars are better left on bicycles. They can be whimsical but seldom handsome.

The Fu Manchu moustache is the epitome of villainy. Closely akin to it are the Simon Legree and the Genghis Khan. The droop and the twirl can be overly melodramatic.

"Spaced" moustaches separate slightly (or exaggeratedly) at the center of the top lip. An individualizing technique, spacing may be simply a matter of brushing outward. In some cases, spacing involves careful clipping, even shaving. The slim vertical line of a spaced moustache tends to split the face in two.

Cropped moustaches may be sparse or dense, yet they're always trimmed in some manner. The most common, acceptable, and non-extreme style, a cropped moustache usually fills the space fully between the nose and upper lip without being too bushy and without any elaborate shaping.

Beard styles vary according to length and the amount of shaping. Disaster strikes when the wrong moustache style accompanies the wrong beard style. Imagine the Fu Manchu with an Amish beard. Quick, turn off the lights.

Except for the Amish beard (when the upper lip is shaven and the jaw is sharply accented by defined shaving), a moustache almost always forms a unity with a beard. Full beards—covering a great deal of

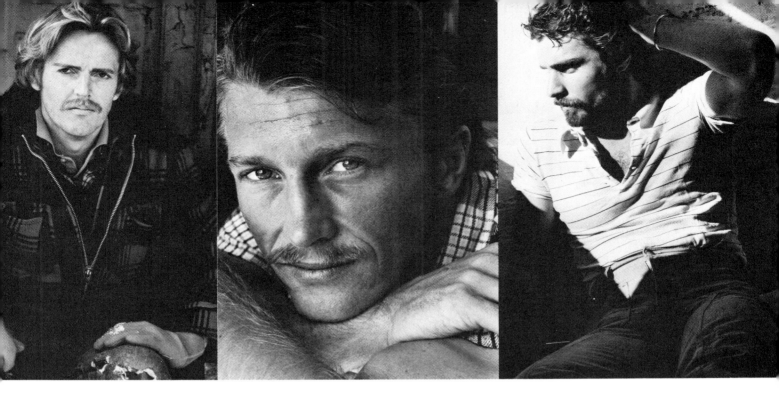

the cheeks, growing from the sideburns and connecting with the moustache while covering the neck at least to the Adam's apple—are the most favored, although the fullness can be either neatly clipped or reminiscent of Saint Nick.

Square beards (with whiskers trimmed in a square from moustache to under the chin but with the rest of the jawline cleanly shaven) and triple tiered beards (when the moustache droops but doesn't join the fringe of beard, which is relegated solely to the lower chin area, with a wisp or tuft of hair beneath the center of the lip) are variations on partial beards. Occasionally partial beards run the risk of looking too self-conscious or prissy. So do elaborate sideburn treatments (see "Side by Side," pages 15–16).

Facial hair shifts facial focus, usually drawing attention to itself at the purposeful expense of other features. On those hard-to-find perfect faces, sane moustaches and/or beards seldom significantly enhance or detract. But for most less fortunate men, growing fringe is a balancing act, rearranging the face into a better perspective.

Unhappily, since facial hair grows as erratically and individualistically as hair atop the head, a guy can't always sprout exactly what he wants. In general, taller men can carry off a lot of hair, not only on the face, but on the head as well. (Very tall and slender men, however, may look better with shorter hair and beards to emphasize their leanness.) Small men are advised to cut beards and moustaches closer to the face. Similarly, the weaker the facial features, the stronger the facial hair can be. In all instances, care must be taken to avoid unflattering results. As with hairstyles, a man may choose to "abstract" himself from the norm by cultivating eccentric styles, but the decision should be purposeful. Whatever the decision, chances are that shaving will still be part of your life; don't miss Chapter 12, "Morning Male: Shaving."

Hair & Life Style

The type of beard or moustache you choose should relate to both your hairstyle and your life-style. If you spend most of your time in a business suit, a wildly woolly beard can make you look like a lumberjack uncomfortable in his Sunday best. Visual clashes are guaranteed to envelop you in a negative image. Appropriateness counts.

A beard doesn't hide a good face. It can accent one

when kept in proportion with the hair on the head, forming a continuation of the hairstyle. Thus, short, neat hair atop demands the symmetry of neat, short hair below.

A period hairstyle and moustache—like the thirties look of sleek hair and thin moustache—can't be done halfway. The moustache could look like a dirty smudge with rampant hair. And the polo image is out of the question with jeans and sneakers; buy a velvet smoking jacket and rent a tuxedo.

Very long hair is almost always well suited to some facial hair to avoid an ethereal effect. A beard will bring the face into focus, halting the hair's distraction from the features. If the beard is overgrown, however, who can see the features for the forest?

Forward Match

Since facial hair should create balance and symmetry, the hairline often dictates what should grow on the lower part of the face. A wide, receding hairline can be counterbalanced with a closely clipped beard and moustache—a far better solution than trying to camouflage the recession. Conversely, narrow foreheads with low hairlines are made more obvious with beards that are too strong. Minimizing the hairline by choosing a short, brushed-from-the-face style and adding a trim moustache can direct attention away from the forehead, balancing the weight of the face. Bald heads are like unpainted canvases; make the face more colorful with a moustache.

Pint Sized

Features too small leave the face looking unanchored. Moustaches give the face ballast by weighting the area between nominal noses and minimal mouths. Nonetheless, the facial hair should be well-trimmed; otherwise underwhelming features are more overwhelmed. Careful shaping and shaving add character to facial hair. Stylized beards, though not necessarily as studied as a Vandyke, may be appropriate.

Pronouncements

Exaggerated features can sometimes be tamed with facial hair since they will appear less emphatic when

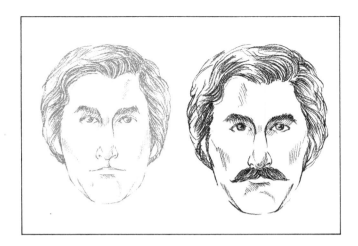

the latter captures the viewer's eye first. Reasonably full moustaches offset largish noses and chins. (However, a jutting chin, if bearded, appears even heavier.) Protruding ears can be underplayed by a moustache alone or, even more camouflaging, with beard and moustache. Moustaches are safer than full beards, since beards, unless they are very crisply groomed, may look extreme. Extreme features plus extreme beards produce sinister effects. If eyebrows are resplendently wild, a bushy moustache or beard compounds the beastliness. It depends on what you're into.

Cheeky

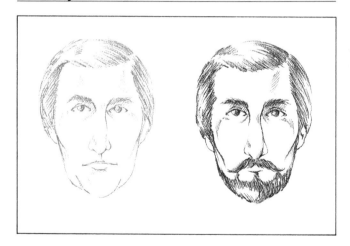

Facial hair adds a new definition to a face. When the cheekbones are next to nonexistent, a moustache is a definite plus. On the other hand, craggy cheekbones with caverns beneath, combined with jagged bone structure, can make a man look terminally ill. Adding a full beard evens out the irregularities. A more individualistic style, even an extraordinary one, makes such a man look decisive, not as if he's in hiding. In some cases, broad faces will appear narrower when a moustache with a tilt, either up or down at the ends, breaks the flatness of the face.

Doubling Up

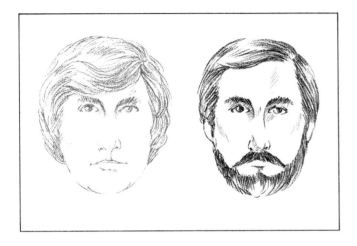

Weak, flabby chins can be offset by the judicious addition of beards, creating semblances of jawlines where none existed. Chubby faces should avoid facial fringes with drawn or shaved-in lines *except* for an emphatic one beneath the chin from earlobes to above the Adam's apple. When hair is styled on the short side and a well-groomed beard is grown and maintained, eyes are framed to better advantage without the distraction of a weak chin. Conversely, a pointy chin is disguised by sprouting a full beard, which visually doubles the chin's size by filling it out and rounding it off.

Attention, Please

Youngish, nondescript faces gain authority and a couple of years with the addition of facial hair. So do faces with pallid coloring. Mr. Bland almost always looks a bit more dashing with fringe benefits. With more men wearing beards and moustaches, adding facial hair won't make you stand out in the crowd, but at least part of your face will gain more prominence.

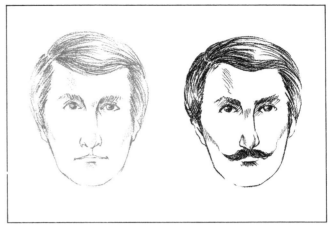

If, however, the beard grows in strangely, get rid of it. Make certain facial hair is a plus, not a minus.

BEWHISKERED
CARING FOR FACIAL HAIR

When facial hair can legitimately be called a moustache or a beard (following the several slow weeks), that's when earnest grooming begins. Naturally, a new beard is kept clean even while it's growing in. Soap and water will probably suffice in the initial stages, but later you'll need shampoo, definitely a mild one that cleans well and leaves the hair soft.

The importance of washing a beard can't be overemphasized. Remember, your face is under it—the same skin that is highly susceptible to eruptions and problems when not properly cleansed. A beard may cover the skin, but it certainly isn't a form of protection. Don't create a bacterial playground at the root of your beard.

If flaking occurs, never use a dandruff shampoo. Such flaking is probably the result of either insufficient rinsing of the beard after shampooing or of not drying the beard correctly. Dampness, after all, is an invitation to bacteria. But don't use blow dryers on beards; the heat is too intense for tender facial skin.

Shampoo the beard away from the face to prevent its coarse texture from irritating the skin.

A beard dries relatively quickly, as the water rolls off. Rubbing a beard dry with a towel usually suffices. Be sure to comb the beard with a wide-toothed comb before tangles set in. Special moustache combs are

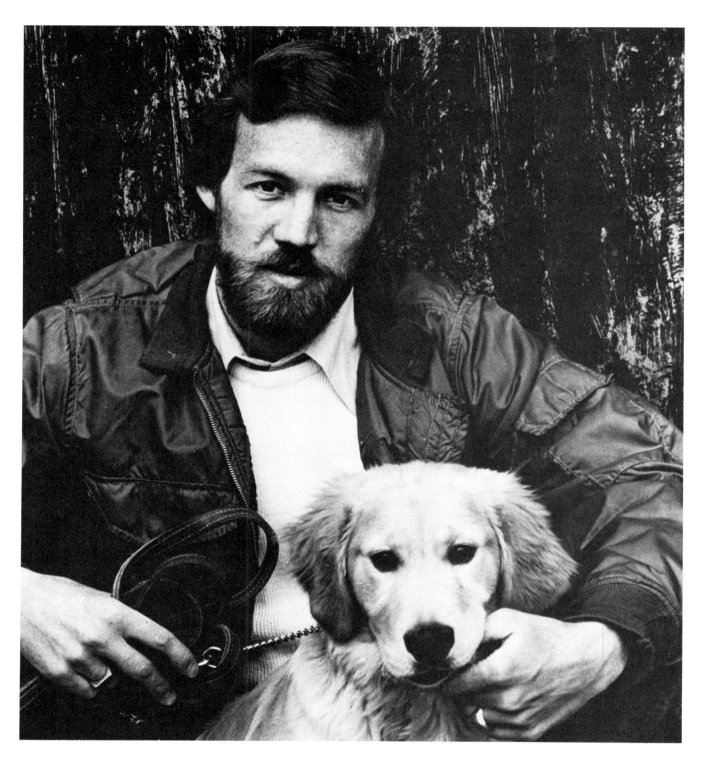

marketed for training and neatening. These are acceptable detanglers, too. Combing should always precede any brushing.

When combing or brushing the beard, do so in the direction you want it to lie. This is almost always a downward motion, with short strokes to round the whiskers along the jaw. Don't use a soft-bristled brush; it can't contend with coarse beard hairs. Although brushing should be firm—moving *through* the beard, not just on its surface—don't be so vigorous that the skin beneath is irritated.

Trimming beards and moustaches is easier when

they're dry, since you can see more clearly what you're clipping away. Soggy, relaxed whiskers have a different shape and appearance than dry ones, making it difficult to gauge what the results will be. Very short moustaches can sometimes be trimmed with toenail clippers.

To trim a full board, brush *up*, comb *out*, loosening the hairs. If the hairs are tangled, remove the knots with your fingers. Rough actions of a comb or brush can break or mangle the hair while irritating the face.

Using a magnifying mirror close up, begin snipping at the tips of the hairs for gentle shaping.

Many experts recommend that scissors and combs be used simultaneously, running the comb through the beard, stopping where you intend to cut, then snipping off the hairs protruding through the teeth of the comb. This is the professional method; it's a good idea to have a pro shape up a beard from time to time. However, many men lack the manual dexterity to maneuver comb and scissors themselves without risking erratic results.

While trimming the beard, it's better to be safe than sorry. If you mistakenly remove too much in one section, the only way to correct the error is to reduce all other areas to the same length. An inherent problem in cutting a beard too short is that the whiskers may curve in, becoming itchy and possibly ingrown.

Trimmers have been specially designed for thinning out a beard. Such devices have razor blades sandwiched between two layers of plastic, with comblike teeth. The instrument is angled and pulled through the hair.

Unfortunately, most trimming-thinning devices perform inconsistently at best. If you use a thinner, take it slow. Heat its blade thoroughly in hot water. Keep it clean.

Some men with light hair find that their facial hair is considerably darker, unattractively so. Using a facial-hair bleach (the type used by women on their upper lips if need be) is not unheard of. This procedure is far safer than bleaching with permanent hair colorings, which are far too harsh. Never do so.

Facial bleaches generally come in complete kits, containing a tube of bleach, a powdered activator, a mixing tray, and a scoop. Ribbons of the bleach cream are squeezed into the mixing tray, then sprinkled with the activator. Using the flat end of a measuring scoop,

mix the cream and powder until completely blended. Now wash your face with soap and *cold* water. Pat dry gently. Apply the mixture to your face with the flat end of the scoop. Spread evenly over the entire area to be lightened. Leave on for fifteen minutes. Remove with the applicator. Rinse your face with cold water. If the hair is not light enough, reapply in the same manner for another ten minutes. Rinse off with cold water.

Be forewarned, however, that if your skin feels sensitive or irritated after application, remove the mixture immediately. Never apply after a hot bath. Open pores increase sensitivity. And for vision's sake, never use facial hair bleaches near the eyes. Should any bleach get in the eyes, rinse out thoroughly with lukewarm water. If stinging persists, see a physician. No one needs a chemical eyewash.

"Paint kits"—permanent coloring dyes self-applied with a paint brush—can lighten or darken beards. Some men have used shoe polish to deepen their beard color. Ridiculous and smudging. Beard and moustache stains are available that are more permanent. But to really do it right, ask your hair stylist to color your beard professionally.

The care and maintenance of a full beard is relatively easy, since proper cleansing and occasional trimming are the extent of the grooming regimen. However, if you decide upon a shaped beard, the demarcation between the shaved and the nonshaved areas must be straight, sharp, and clean. Shaving must be superclose (see Chapter 12). Ditto for a moustache versus the nonhairy cheeks and chin.

Should your fringe appear dry—yes, it can happen here, too—take care how you overcome the problem. Hair tonics or creams can be *sparingly* used. An oily beard is even less appealing that oily hair. Your best bet is to investigate good conditioning shampoos.

Don't rub aftershave lotion or cologne into a beard or moustache. These products are alcohol based, causing whiskers to dry, robbing them of their naturally protective oils.

If you're unhappy with a full beard or even a lengthy moustache and want to be rid of it, first remove most of the hair with scissors before shaving. When this step is omitted, razor pull can be too great, leading to a severe abrasion on your face.

CHAPTER 9

WEATHER VAIN

SEASONAL CONSIDERATIONS

Even hermits occasionally surface for air. More gregarious men usually spend at least portions of their days in the unpredictable environment of the outside world. Just as no true year-round wardrobes exist away from the heat-drenched Equator or the ice-bound Ples, the same hair care regimen can't stand up to all weather conditions.

THE FRIENDLY SKIES
SPRING & FALL

The comparative mildness of the spring and fall seasons treat hair most kindly. If hair has been neglected during the previous season's more extreme onslaught, it must first be repaired before it can enjoy the friendly skies.

For different reasons, both winter and summer may cause hair to become drier and more brittle. When fairer weather arrives, normalcy reasserts itself. At least it should. New hair growth may be fine and dandy. But what about the abused hair attached to the healthy regrowth? At the beginning of the spring and fall seasons you might need to saturate the ends of the hair daily with an appropriate conditioner, perhaps a mild balsam type. Pour the conditioner into your palms, and using small circular motions, gently rub into the ends of your hair over the entire head. Don't push down to the scalp. Let the conditioner sit on the hair tips for a few minutes. Think beautiful or wicked thoughts. Now rinse thoroughly. Towel dry. Comb into place. Wait until all remaining moisture has evaporated before going outside.

This technique controls split ends (the consequence of severe dryness) and lubricates the outer problem portions of the hair shafts. Condition the entire head of hair about once a week. After a few weeks, the situation should be under control. When you have your hair styled, the damaged ends will be clipped away. Now take sufficient care to prevent any new abuse.

For the bulk of the benign weather, follow a normal

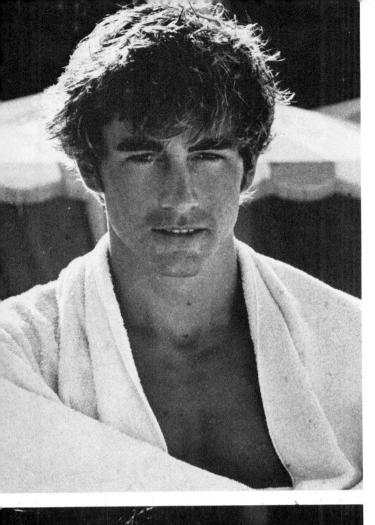
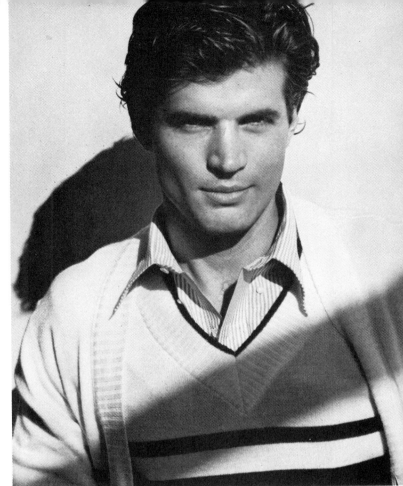
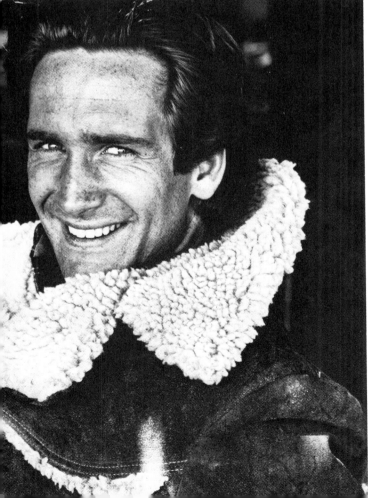
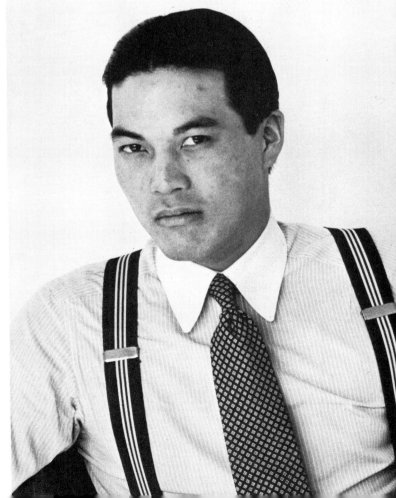

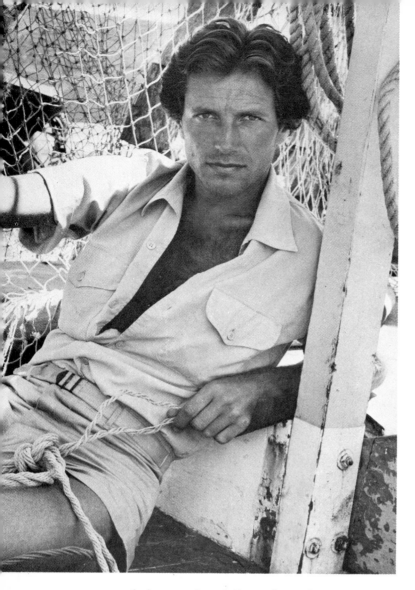

course of shampooing daily and conditioning as required.

Toward the end of these seasons, you should take some precautionary steps to prepare the hair for either winter's chilling blasts or summer's harsh rays. Massage the scalp longer to stimulate circulation. Condition more often, since any slight hair problem will be heightened during the hardy months.

Toward the end of spring is the best time to use a lifter, one of those coloring agents that lightens the hair by only a shade or two while brightening and conditioning it. Color weaving also anticipates some of the bleaching that occurs from exposure to the summer sun. On the other hand, if your hair naturally bleaches out easily but you don't want it to, a neutral henna treatment during spring's closing days will protect the hair and help you maintain your natural color when summer begins.

Spring and fall are good seasons to try new hairstyles. Nature is changing, why shouldn't you?

THE COLD WAR
WINTER

A widespread misconception is that when temperatures drop, so should daily shampooing. Wrong, unless your hair is exceedingly dry. Keeping hair its cleanest is more important when the wind starts whistling: Central heating and external pollution conspire together to make improperly cleansed hair look lifelessly lackadaisical. The answer is maintaining the shampooing frequency while increasing conditioning frequency. Stimulating scalp massage should also be augmented, since the entire body, including its oil production and blood circulation, tends to be more sluggish when temperatures plummet.

Cold-war propaganda also states that hair should always be covered when exposed to the cold. True, harsh and windy weather does dry the hair, particularly when the humidity is low. On the other hand, unventilated headwear, especially felt hats, stimulate perspiration that can breed bacteria. Knitted caps are far better, since air can circulate. Yet, for some unknown reason, it appears that fresh air—even fresh frigid air—aids in healthy hair growth. Hardhats, then, should treat their hair to a half-hour sun and air bath every day, whatever the thermometer reads. So should everybody else. A brisk, hatless walk also helps maintain muscle tone at a time when we're usually more sedentary.

Since low humidity does rob moisture from the hair, buying a humidifier is one defense. So is spraying on a pre-blow-drying protector if you use moisture-reducing dryers or stylers to keep your hair in shape. Some presprays can be used instead of hair conditioners. They also help hold the style.

Guys with moustaches who sometimes discover dry patches under or near their fringes due to improper rinsing should be advised that cold weather can aggravate the situation—even if it went unnoticed during milder times. Since moustaches and beards become drier during winter, using hair lotions on them might be stepped up a bit. Usually facial hair should be grown longer in winter, since hairstyles are often longer. Longer doesn't mean wilder. Denser beards require more shaping, not less.

FATHERLY SUN ADVICE

SUMMER

Intense sun strips the hair of natural oils. For men with oily hair, summer does them a favor. But fellows whose hair is usually normal may experience new problems, and guys with dry hair definitely will, if measures aren't taken to protect hair from abuse.

Covering the hair with a cap is one alternative. But as we've seen, tightly fitting hats that don't allow the scalp to breathe increase scalp perspiration. Profuse sweating, which is more likely in summer anyway, makes fine hair look stringy, thick hair a mess. Straw hats or Panamas are protective, while permitting air to circulate, but their brims can create some unexpected and unwanted bumps. Wearing them can also mat the hair.

One notion many hair stylists promote is rubbing an ample amount of hair conditioner through the hair and leaving it there before spending prolonged periods in the sun. Obviously the hair will look rather greasy. This oily, wet look appears more purposeful when the hair is slicked back off the face. Should the conditioner dry away or be removed as a result of swimming, applying more conditioner—the same way you apply more suntan lotion and perhaps at the same time—is the recommendation.

Naturally, the conditioner should be shampooed out of the hair when you leave the beach, since the oils in the conditioner attract airborne debris. After shampooing you needn't condition again. Two tablespoons of vinegar diluted in a cup of lukewarm water will close the hair cuticles. So will lemon juice sluiced through the hair.

Speaking of lemons, don't rub them on your hair to promote sun-bleaching. The results are at best erratic.

Also, citrus essences (limes more so than lemons) can photosensitize the skin, causing burns.

Tropical humidity can cause porous, wavy hair to curl and swell. Light hair dressings help a bit, but greasy ones run when you perspire. Plastering with hair spray looks bad any time but worst in summer: Easy living is best reflected in easier, more casual hairstyles. Shorter lengths, of course, make summer hair care easier. And that includes facial hair as well. Beards and moustaches warm up the underlying skin during hot spells. Keeping them more neatly and closely cropped permits more ventilation and decreases perspiration. Splashing beards and moustaches with water from time to time is another cooling touch.

Summer humidity may turn thick, kinky hair tighter, because damp air and perspiration can shrink the curls into knots. Relaxed perming gives a consistently looser look. Fine, dense hair requiring extensive blow drying to shape it up is also easier to control when permed. Straight hair that hangs limp and becomes flat in summer heat likewise receives a lift from body perming. As noted, however, permanent restructuring robs hair of some moisture, so extra conditioning will then be on the summer agenda. On the positive side, curly hair is quick and easy, with fingers the best styling tools. Sane color changes can add texture and body to lifeless or dull hair, while starting you on your way to faded glory. Since the sun bleaches unevenly, color weaving comes closest to looking natural.

Since you're more likely to shampoo twice a day during the summer, try the trick of diluting your shampoo with an equal part of water before washing your hair. Harsh products are exactly what your hair doesn't need when it's constantly under attack from the elements. Spritzing the hair periodically throughout the day with a mist of water quenches its thirst. But don't drench it.

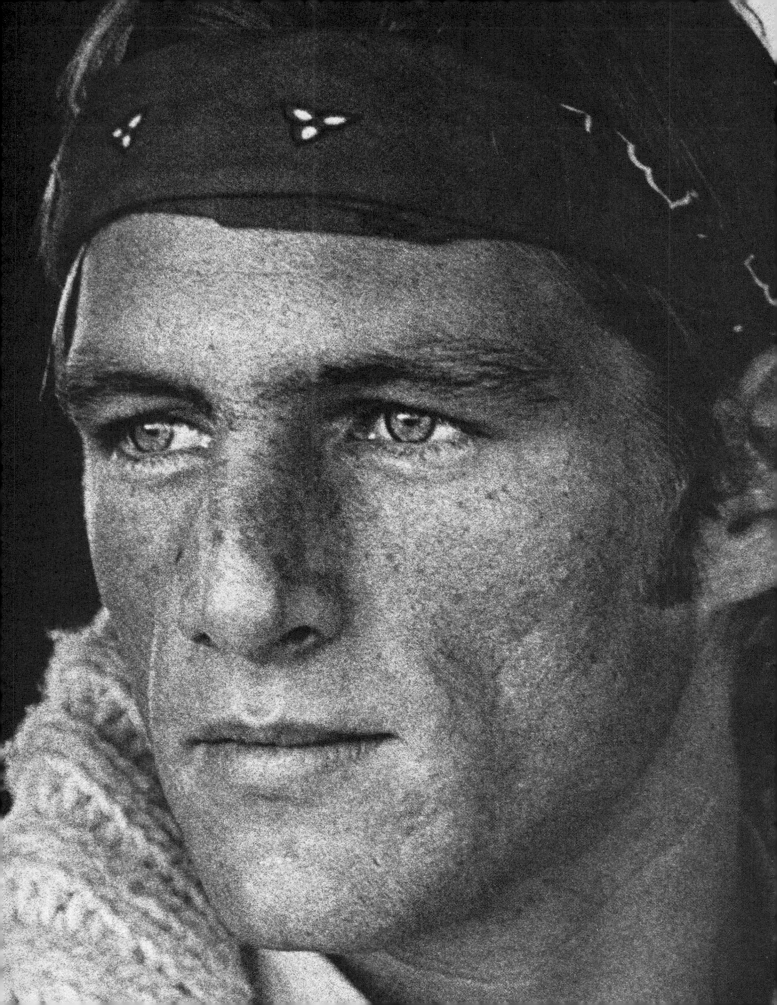

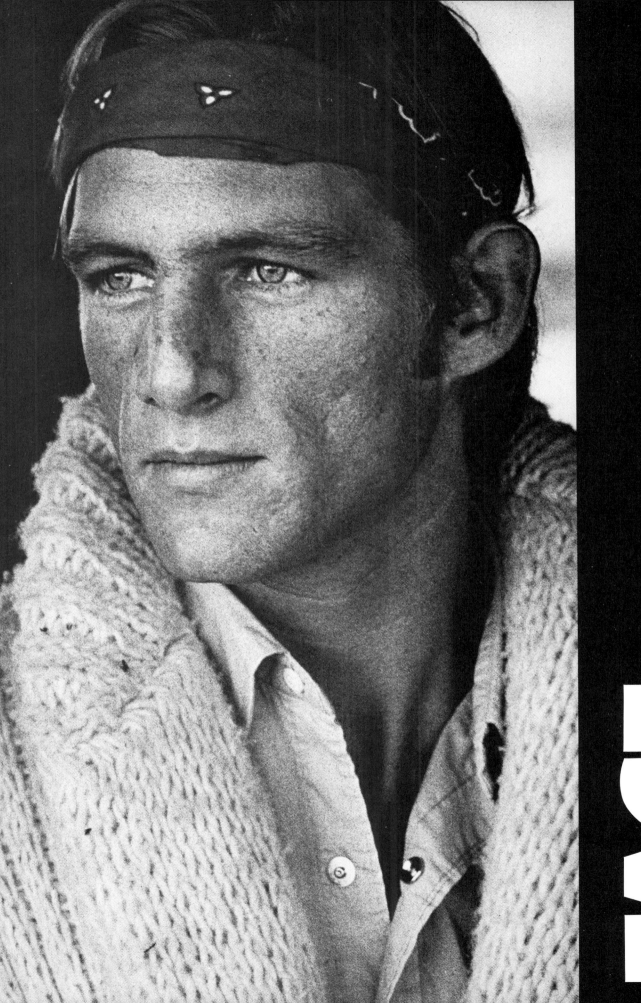

FACE

CHAPTER 10

CLEAN LIVING
SKIN CARE

Probably as many hypotheses for skin care exist as supposed cures for the common cold, and most are just as suspect. But one fact is undeniable: Since most men don't wear foundation or makeup of any kind, with our constantly exposed faces, we require as much—or more—skin assistance as the distaff side. Not that we need to spend as much or more time, energy, and money than they, heaven forbid.

CELL BLOCKS
SKIN STRUCTURE

Look at yourself in a mirror. Hopefully your face seems vital and alive. Ironically, the cells that comprise the skin's surface are dead. How's that for happy news?

Skin is divided into two layers. The outer, visible one (epidermis) is protective, creating a barrier against harmful substances in the environment. Flattened, dead cells bind together as a resilient, waterproof surface ever in the process of being rubbed, washed, or scaled away. Deep in the epidermis is the basal cell layer, where new cells are constantly being produced. These migrate to the surface of the skin and will eventually also be shed.

Beneath the epidermis is the skin's invisible inner layer (dermis) that supports and nourishes the outer layer. The dermis cannot regenerate itself, so if injured, permanent scarring results. When the connective fibers between the outer and the inner layers break down or lose their elasticity, wrinkles set in.

Housed within the dermis are various oil-producing and sweat glands, plus hair follicles, all of which are connected to the skin's surface via tubular ducts.

Sebaceous glands (the technical name for oil-producing glands) are especially significant in the skin's appearance. These glands produce an oily-fatty substance called sebum for lubrication and protec-

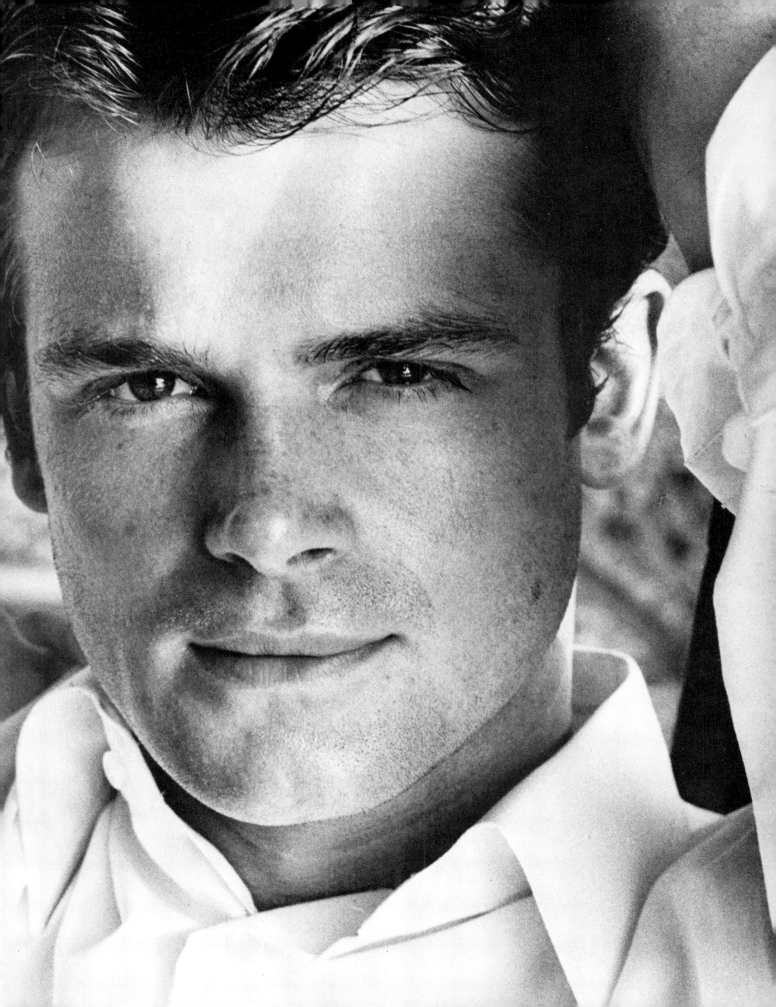

tion of the organism. The amount of sebum secreted affects the degree of oiliness of the skin and hair. Since the sebaceous glands are influenced by androgenic (male) hormones, sebum production starts pumping during puberty and continues throughout the life-span, lessening with old age. This partially explains why the skin becomes drier in later years.

Sweat glands regulate the body's temperature and eliminate internal waste material through the skin.

The skin is more concentrated with nerve endings than the rest of the body. These make the skin sensitive to heat, cold, pain, and touch.

In addition to serving as a covering for the body, skin protects internal tissues from the sun by producing melanin, a dark pigment that absorbs the harmful ultraviolet rays in a phenomenon known as tanning. It also thickens when exposed to the sun.

Acting as a shield, the skin is impervious to most substances that, if introduced directly into the system, would wreak havoc. Ironically, many claims for cosmetics assert that the products "penetrate" the skin. Fortunately, they don't. These concoctions *may* be slightly absorbed into the epidermis if they have a high percentage of water, since water is the only known substance that will actually be ingested by the skin naturally. This only takes place within the outer, dead cells. If artificial steps are not taken to "lock in" the moisture, it will simply evaporate.

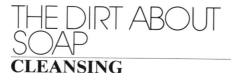

THE DIRT ABOUT SOAP
CLEANSING

Because body wastes and oils are excreted through the skin's pores onto its surface and because atmospheric pollution gravitates there too, thorough cleansing is much more than a cosmetic consideration: Only clean skin is healthy skin. Since the face is constantly exposed (and judged by others), it is understandably the correct focus for a major amount of grooming efforts.

Skin, especially facial skin, comes under the influences of geography, season, age, and general health, plus personal care. Involved in personal care are procedures some specialists call preventive

measures, simply meaning that what a man does earlier may prevent deterioration later. This advice can only be taken on faith, for most fellows aren't equipped with a crystal ball, let alone one that can foresee the consequences of alternate routes. Although individual skin characteristics must be weighed in developing a personal care regimen for the face, the mechanics of good cleansing must first be explored.

As mentioned, collecting on the skin's surface is a motley assortment of decomposed cells, sweat, oil, waste, bacteria, pollutants, and other no-goodies that can clog the pores. If the buildup of dead cells is not shed, this, too, leads to blocked and enlarged pores. The skin becomes thicker and looks coarser. Cleansing alone isn't enough to solve all the potential problems, but it is the correct starting point.

Many men cleanse haphazardly, splashing a little soap and water on the face, barely rinsing, then toweling dry. The dirt isn't totally removed, and joining the facial debris is now another unwelcome guest—residual soap that also helps clog the pores while drawing moisture from the possibly already dessicated dead cells.

The most important task of a cleanser—whether it's soap, cream, lotion, or liquid—is to remove as much dirt and oil from the skin as possible without irritating it. (Some potent acids could remove *all* the dirt and *all* the skin, too.) Ideally, a cleanser should also be completely removable, either with water or another means not too difficult or time-consuming.

In most instances, old-fashioned soap and water meet these requirements best. But some soaps are good, some fair-to-middling, and some bad for the face. For men with extra-dry skin, any kind of soap may be harmful.

To begin with, not all soaps are "soap." For centuries, real soap has been made from similar formulations of water, sodium salts, and fatty acids, plus variouis oils (some only to enhance sudsing). More modern in formula, *detergent* soap is really "soapless" in that chemicals have replaced the various natural ingredients to achieve the same results: loosening the dead cells, cutting through the oils, and dislodging the dirt so that unwanted substances can be rinsed away. Detergent soaps aren't necessarily harsh (but they can be); they're just not true "soap." Whereas the real thing leaves a gooky bathtub ring, detergent soaps seldom do.

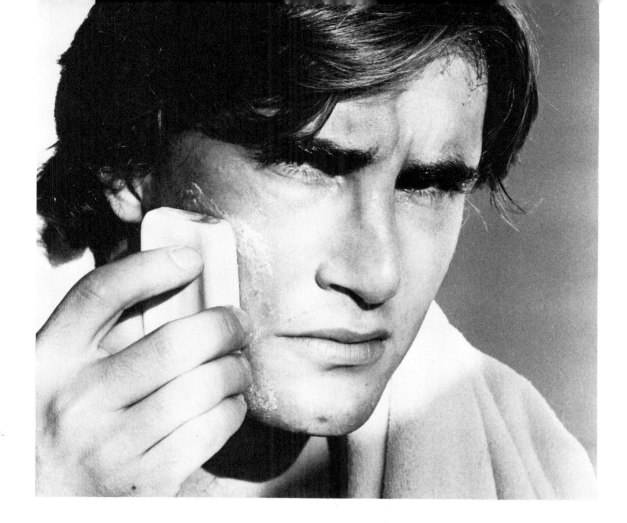

Real soaps can be *deodorant soaps*, which enlist antibacterial agents to check body odor (the face isn't subject to this problem, so such additives are unnecessary and possibly dangerous for facial skin); *Castile soaps*, made with olive oil instead of fat; *cocoa butter soaps*, made with their namesake instead of fat; *fruit soaps*, with essences or compounds dubious for cleansing although adding an unusual fragrance and feel; *clear soaps*, created by a process that makes them more soluble by increasing the fat content and adding alcohol, glycerine, and perhaps sugar; *superfatted soaps*, which as their name suggests have a substantially greater ratio of fat (which lessens their effectiveness in removing fats and oils since some residue generally remains on the skin); *cream soaps*, which add some cold cream or a similar extra ingredient to the soap (making the soap slightly less efficient for cleansing, although cream soaps supposedly are milder than many other soaps); and *true soaps*, unperfumed, uncolored, un-anythinged other than simply "soap." To repeat, not all soaps are the same.

In addition to soaps, an apparent myriad of other facial cleansers are currently being offered.

Reputedly formulated by the Greek physician Galen about *A.D.* 150, *cold cream* — then a mixture of loads of water, olive oil, beeswax, and rose petals — is the basis of all modern cleansing creams. More primitive in origin but still occasionally employed are oils and greases such as animal, vegetable, and mineral oils to wipe away surface dirt. (How anyone knows this is mind-boggling, but cavemen, when they wanted to spruce up, just rubbed their faces and bodies with bear fat.)

Cold creams and these oils liquefy on the warm skin to loosen and suspend foreign particles. When they are toweled or tissued away, a greasy residue remains. This can be removed with soap and water or an alcohol-based astringent (a clear liquid product usually promoted for oily skin to "refreshen" it).

Most of the ingredients in *cleansing creams* resemble those in cold creams, but these cleansers are bolstered with additional ones (often alcohol) to make them thinner and lighter. Cleansing creams feel less oily than conventional cold creams but also leave some filmy residue on the face.

Cleansing lotions are even thinner and usually come in liquid form, but a little leftover residue may still cling.

Rinsable cleansers are primarily lotions containing small amounts of soap or soaplike substances. The formulas are modified so they can be removed completely by dousing the face with water, which won't remove regular creams. As such, rinsable cleansers work very much like soap and water, since any residue can be splashed away without resorting to an additional step. However, rinsable cleansers usually don't foam. No matter; they still work niftily.

Cold creams and the assorted traditional cleansing oils and lotions are almost never irritating to the skin. However, as noted, they may not cleanse as thoroughly as soap and water or rinsable cleansers, and they do have the disadvantage of clinging to the skin. On the other hand, although soaps and rinsable cleansers clean better, they are potentially more irritating to the skin. This danger increases the longer they are in contact with the skin. Obviously, then, when such soaps are used, cleansing should be rapid and rinsing extra cautious. Overcleansing and insufficient removal are the real threats.

For optimum results, the face should first be thoroughly wetted with warm water. If soap is the vehicle, it should be lathered on the palms and rubbed quickly onto the damp face with the fingertips. If a liquid cleanser is employed, the face should still first be completely wetted before following the label directions. Three to four complete rinsings with fresh water are an extra insurance.

Recognizing that the alkaline nature of soap and soaplike substances may be irritating, some companies have developed *pH- (or acid-) balanced soaps and cleansers*. A word of explanation is required.

Actually, pH is not a magic ingredient but the measurement of hydrogen ion concentration. Expressed more simply, the pH factor is the relative degree of acidity or alkalinity in a product. Not describing a product's ingredients, it measures whether the resulting combination is neutral, acidic, or alkaline.

Why bother? Because studies indicate that normal, healthy skin (or hair) is slightly acidic. However, the skin itself isn't really being measured. Rather, the acidity comes from the secretions (sebum, in particular) which normally form an invisible (and, unfortunately, occasionally a very visible) film on the face. This is called the skin's acid mantle and is generally thought to be protective as well as lubricating. By bolstering cleansers so that their degree of acidity corresponds to the acid mantle, companies theorize that their products will not be disruptive to the skin.

The theory sounds reasonable. However, it ignores the fact that the pH of the skin (or scalp or hair) varies not only with the individual but also in different parts of the body of the same individual and at different times in the same parts of the same individual. Also, when the pH for one reason or another is artificially altered, the body will return to its usual pH, unassisted, within a few hours.

Likewise, even makers of pH-balanced products concede that cleansers so formulated aren't necessarily good. The ingredients and other "balancings" must be evaluated.

So where does that leave the man out to find how best to cleanse his face? Is he left perpetually dangling midair? Not necessarily. But before he can make a commonsense decision, some other factors must still be explored.

Don't throw your hands up in disgust! Calm down! No one ever said that looking good was easy. Simple advice is often simplistic. Good grooming is a series of interrelated steps. Skip one and the whole regimen is thrown off balance. That's why the choice of a good facial cleanser revolves around what additional steps will be undertaken.

PORE BOY
SCRUBS

After a man reaches maturity, cleansing alone may not remove the face's dead outer cells fast enough. Although well-cared-for skin may never be so inclined, sometimes the adult face may appear coarse and sallow, increasingly so as the years mount. Even proper moisturizing efforts may not prove sufficient.

In such instances, "thinning"—hastening the removal of the dead surface with an abrasive of some kind—may be the remedy for leathery-looking skin.

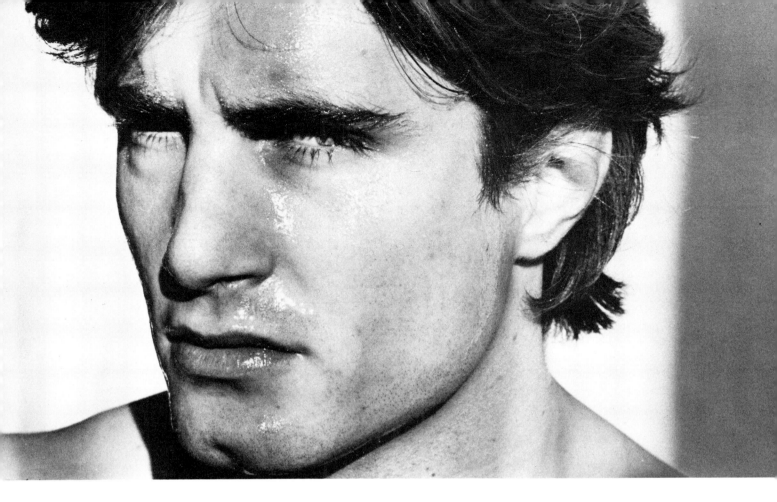

(This type of self-administered thinning should not be confused with chemical thinners, which induce peeling of the skin, primarily a medical technique.)

By shaving daily, a man in effect is thinning part of his face. But unshaved areas, like the forehead and nose, may also need thinning. In general, thinned skin feels smoother, is more translucent, and has a healthier glow.

Sponges, even rough washcloths, serve as mechanical thinners for the face, but with limited effectiveness. *Abrasive cleansers* are rougher on the skin, thus removing more dead cells. These cleansers come in two types: as soaps with hard particles milled into the bar; or as beads or grains dispersed in liquid, lotion, or gel bases. For ease, since they work the same way, they can be lumped together as *scrubs*.

Scrubs work by abrading the skin with these tiny particles in order to rub away the dead cells. This should never be done daily. Certain dermatologists suggest using scrubs twice a week, regardless of skin type. However, if skin is tender or sensitive, this practice can be uncomfortable, not to say downright ir-

ritating. Scrub too hard and you'll bleed. The eye areas should always be avoided since skin is thinnest there.

Even hale and hearty skin is more vulnerable after thinning. It is more easily sunburned, for example, because some of the protective pigment has been ground away in the process. The face may be slightly inflamed. A protective moisturizer is essential after thinning. For these reasons, it is very difficult to advise whether or not a man must thin his face. Be very gentle if experimenting.

FRESH FACE
ASTRINGENTS

A group of products called fresheners, toners, and astringents is sold principally as a secondary boost to cleansing. In some cases, such as when you are using oils or creams that leave a residue on the face, these liquids complete the removal job.

To some extent, the three terms are interchangeable, although the alcoholic content presumably increases from fresheners to toners to astringents. But alcohol is the most important ingredient in all of them.

Alcohol works as a degreaser and de-oiler. Most men are unaware that a major active ingredient in aftershaves is alcohol, so they, too, can perform as astringents, albeit expensive ones. On the other hand, diluting rubbing alcohol with water (or using it straight) will also work.

Astringents are most often applied with cotton balls to a freshly washed face to finalize the cleansing process. But they can also be used to remove moisturizers or merely to whisk away oil from prone zones such as the nose or forehead at any time of the day without resorting to complete cleansing.

Although some claims are made that astringents reduce the size of the pores, they don't. However, they can make the pores look slightly smaller by helping to unclog them. Similarly, these lotions may mildly irritate the skin (causing it to puff up a bit), which also makes the pores appear smaller, although the effect soon dissipates.

Since alcohol reportedly tends to dry the skin, some specialists say astringents should only be used by oily-skin sufferers. Naturally, others say the complete opposite, recommending that unless the skin is very, very dry, astringents should be applied every evening at bedtime following the primary cleanser for the most rigorous and thorough cleansing possible.

As with cleansers, suggested use or nonuse will depend upon what other steps are included in a fellow's skin care program. This topic will be outlined according to skin type more precisely later in this chapter.

WATER PROOF
MOISTURIZING

Repeating the fact that the outer layer of the skin is dead may seem ghoulish, but the reminder is central to understanding the steps crucial to good skin care.

When the new (and living) cells are produced in the basal membrane at the bottom of the epidermis, they are plump and moist with water. (Like the earth's surface, the human body is largely water.) But these rotund little rascals start losing moisture almost immediately, so by the time they've completed their journey to the outside world, they are flat and practically water-free. Only one substance will puff them up again—water. And since the dead cells can't drill any wells to summon up extra moisture faster from beneath the skin, the water supply must be replenished externally. When it isn't, those dead cells prove that they're dead by lacking any sign of vitality. Dull and literally lifeless, they lie around until sloughed. But the newer cells replacing them look and are just as dead by the time they surface. With only a slight pun intended, water is life-giving to our dead skin.

Many types of products are promoted as moisturizers when they aren't. Technically, they're often emollients, which means softeners. They keep the skin softer by retarding water evaporation from the skin. Water, then, is the true moisturizer. Tests have proved that soaking removed dead skin in oils or greases or what-have-you won't soften it, although even a drop of water will be absorbed and start softening the skin almost immediately. However, left to its own devices, without the addition of a substance to hold the moisture in, that old dead skin will give up its ghost once more by letting the water evaporate.

The naturally secreted oils of the skin form a barrier to retard water evaporation, but these oils are removed during the cleansing process. And they *should* be, since they have been intermixed with other harmful substances. After cleansing, some new barrier should replace the body's own. Some say that oily skins need a new protector too, since their problem is too much oil, not too much water in the skin. For men with dry skin, the body has definitely constructed an inadequate barrier to begin with. Although the body will naturally replace this protective film in a time, much-needed moisture may possibly be lost in the meantime.

The working of any evaporation-inhibitor is the same whether the moisturizing product's price is cheap or princely. These inhibitors do not enter the skin to any extent. Ingredients that are insoluble in water—oil or cream—are dispersed in the moisturizer so that, when applied, they rest on the skin, depositing a film to imprison the moisture beneath.

Moisturizers should only be applied to a freshly cleansed face. Since their function is to trap as much moisture as possible, they are even more effective if rubbed onto the face while it is damp. One Hollywood makeup man suggests dousing the face with a mini-

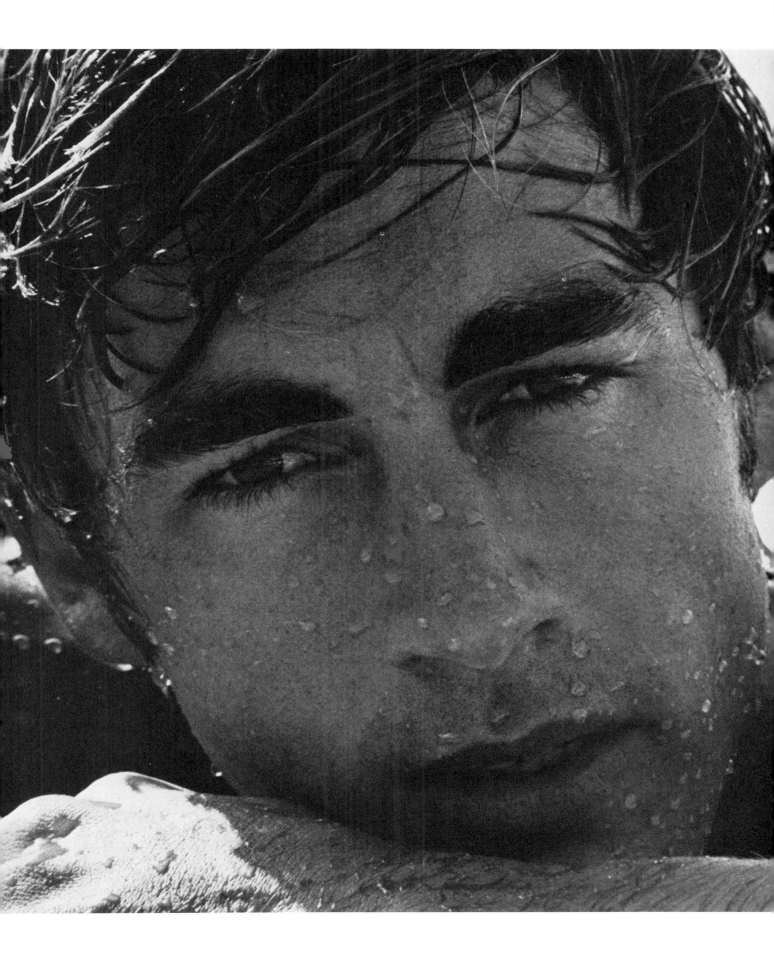

mum of thirty handsful of water before spreading on a moisturizer.

Although most men shy away from using moisturizers, they shouldn't. Skin is skin; it doesn't know if it's male or female, poor thing. Any gendered skin needs protection, meaning a moisturizer.

CLEARLY EVIDENT
NORMAL SKIN

Nobody's perfect, and few, if any, men have perfect facial skin. Normal skin is a type best described by what it isn't: It isn't dry or oily, blemished or sensitive, dull or constantly blushing. The pores aren't enlarged, nor are they too small, and there are no crepelike lines. All in all, the skin looks, well, normal.

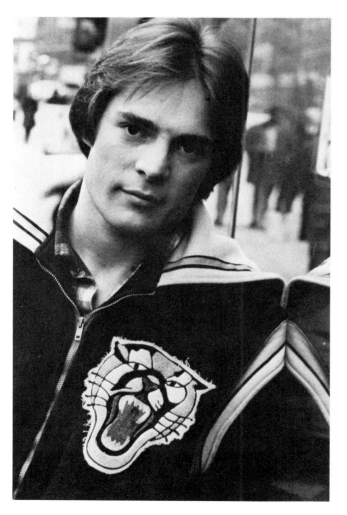

As mentioned, the sebum produced by the sebaceous glands affects the dryness or oiliness of the skin. Men with normal skin secrete enough sebum to lubricate and protect their faces, no more nor less. Cleansing can't control the amount of sebum produced but will affect its visibility. Even normal skin, when uncleansed for a day or two, will look greasy. On the other hand, overcleansing may remove too much oil too often, permitting more moisture evaporation and courting dryness.

Is this too theoretical? If skin is presently normal, someone's doing something right. Why tamper with success? Yet, over the long view, normal skin today may not be so normal tomorrow, so a man should consider the following points to determine if he wants to persist in his current skin care regimen or if he should alter it.

Cleansing: Washing the face twice a day, in the morning before shaving and in the evening before going to bed, will suffice under normal circumstances. Soap and water, the most efficient and effective method, should not be irritating if a moisturizing film is applied after cleansing to lock in always-welcome water.

If from perverse vanity a man associates moisturizing with effeminancy (a misguided notion) and therefore refuses to do so (a pigheaded decision), he needs to get his head together.

Scrubs: These skin abrasives to hasten the removal of dead cells by rubbing them off are controversial. Not to be used indiscriminately, they may not be needed by a man with normal skin, at least during his twenties and thirties, perhaps never. If the skin tone looks especially dull but otherwise the skin is normal, resorting to scrubs from time to time might be advisable but only when the blahs are persistent. Then scrubs replace an occasional bedtime cleansing.

Astringents: Their value is likewise dubious for a man with normal skin, unless his cleanser isn't water-rinsable. If the skin is normal tending toward oiliness, then a third washing per day (followed by proper moisturization) could eliminate any need for astringents. However, if prepackaged astringent pads are used midday to degrease the nose and forehead, and if applying another bit of moisturizer is impossible afterward, the face should be splashed with abundant water and "dried" with the palms. At least the outer skin surface will be superficially replenished for a while.

Moisturizing: Ideally, whenever the skin's natural protection is removed, it should be replaced. Morning moisturizing should complete the morning shave. For some unknown and ungodly reason, many men like the stinging slap from an aftershave splashed on their raw faces. Perhaps the jolt seems manly. But aftershave lotions can also be somewhat drying, while aftershave balms can be more soothing. If a man insists upon dousing his dewhiskered skin with conventional aftershaves, so be it. Naturally, he now must incorporate another step in his skin routine: rinsing away the aftershave with loads of lukewarm water, splashed not only on the razed areas but over the entire face. Leaving the face damp, he should now apply some type of moisturizer in any manner he fancies. Generally, water-based moisturizers spread more easily and seldom look greasy. The moisturizer should be allowed to dry on the face. Although no telltale signs should divulge its presence, if too much has been inadvertently applied, the residue can be tissued away.

If an aftershave balm is used in lieu of lotion, it can simply be applied to the damp face that has been thoroughly rinsed after shaving. It needn't be splashed away and will eliminate adding an extra moisturizing step. In fact, the same aftershave balm can be used as a moisturizer at bedtime following cleansing. However, less expensive preparations will work just as well.

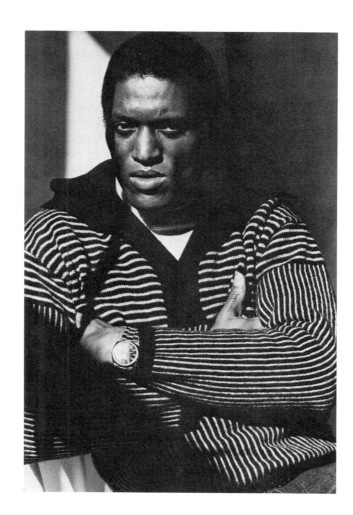

SHINING EXAMPLE
OILY SKIN

It's generally assumed that men, especially black men, have oilier skin than women. Perhaps, but there's no hard evidence and no logical reason that this is so. Why some oil-producing glands are overactive isn't clear. The main concern for men with oily skin should be removing the excess without removing too much moisture. Yet oiliness is subjective. Unclean normal skin, even dry skin, may appear oily. Some areas, like the nose, are endowed with more sebaceous glands and assume an oily aspect more easily.

Generally, oily skin is characterized by enlarged pores and an almost ever-present "glide" to the skin. If after waking in the morning, a man rubs a piece torn from a paper bag across his forehead and the paper turns translucent, that's a shining example of oiliness.

Cleansing: Some dermatologists insist that even oily-skinned men should only wash their faces twice a day, at retiring and when rising. They cite moisture loss as their rationale. However, if steps are taken to rehydrate the skin, why shouldn't a fellow wash his oily face three, four, five times a day? Unchecked oily skin attracts pollutants from the air like a magnet and courts problems. Old-fashioned soap and water degrease and de-oil swiftly and easily. Cream soaps, cocoa butter soaps, superfatted varieties, and the like all leave a residue, so they should be avoided.

Scrubs: Often, but not necessarily, cellular buildup is more rapid on oily skin, and it can be quite tenacious. Since the pores are usually enlarged to accommodate the constant pumping of sebum, they also can be more easily clogged with debris that might not otherwise gain entrance into smaller pores. Thinning scrubs therefore make more sense for men with oily skin than for any other complexion. Their abrasive particles help unclog blocked pores while accelerating the sloughing of dead cells that cause the skin to appear leathery or coarse. But because scrubs are far from gentle, thinning more than two or three times a week is unwise. Astringents shouldn't be applied onto the raw, thinned skin. In fact, some type of soothing moisturizer (nonoily, of course) should complete the thinning. For obvious reasons, scrubs are bedtime procedures, never to be attempted before shaving.

Astringents: Men with oily skin can use astringents after cleansing to ensure that all soap has been removed and to whisk away any oils that might remain within the pores. Astringents can also be used throughout the day to rid newly surfacing oils. The problem with alcohol astringents used extravagantly is that the skin's surface can become dehydrated even though the overall condition is oily. Thus, it's better to wash the face, use an astringent, then to moisturize lightly than it is to use an astringent without rehydrating and moisturizing. If it's impracticable to do the whole thing, remember that splashing water on the face after using an astringent and "palming" the face dry is better than nothing. Being primarily alcohol, astringents evaporate quickly, so their performance isn't diluted by water after they've done their job of removing oils from the face and pores. As noted, aftershave lotions can be used as astringents, and so can plain rubbing alcohol.

Moisturizing: Ever notice how the face of someone with oily skin may occasionally look rough and flaky, supposedly the classic symptoms of dry skin? That's because too much water has been lost from the skin's surface from extra usage of soap and astringents. Too creamy or oily moisturizers aren't solutions, since when the sebum eventually surfaces and mixes with the protector, the skin will appear even oilier. Fortunately, as written earlier, a moisturizer needn't be thick to work.

OIL EMBARGO
DRY SKIN

Because the skin's oil production decreases with age, dry skin is usually associated with old age. But

for numerous reasons, men can suffer prematurely from dry skin. Constant exposure to the sun and elements contributes to dryness. So does improper care, especially the failure to moisturize protectively. But sebaceous glands producing insufficient amounts of sebum to guard the skin against moisture loss is the major cause of persistently dry skin. The pores are very small, and the surface is often flaky. Happily, dry skin attracts less airborne debris and usually doesn't become as dirty as normal or oily skin. Nonetheless, for health reasons it must still be cleansed. Unhappily, cleansing compounds the dry condition by further reducing the meager amount of moisture in the skin. Attention must be paid.

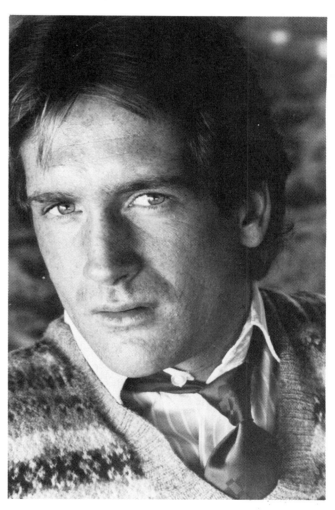

Cleansing: If so-called specialists disagree on other subjects, they are positively at loggerheads about how best to cleanse dry skin. Some dogmatically decree that since soap and water have passed the test of time, they're still what should be used. Others retort,

"Never!" A man with dry skin faces some tough decisions that only he can make. He must weigh cleansing efficiency and thoroughness against comfort and appearance.

For dry-skinned men, the steps following cleansing are more telltale for the skin's appearance than washing is. One regimen is not very complicated: Wash every morning with pure soap and water, splashing like crazy to rinse away all lather, then splashing even more. Next, shave, either with an electric razor or, if with a blade, by first smoothing a small amount of facial cream onto the wet face before adding shaving foam; then, after waiting a minute or so to ensure softening and wetting of the beard, shave; start splashing water again like an exuberant seal, removing *every* trace of shaving foam. (After using an electric razor, do the seal trick anyway; it feels good.) While the face is still wet, apply a moisturizer. At bedtime, save face with a rinsable cleanser, splash, and moisturize. If you're not man enough to try a cleanser, then probably cold cream also carries a stigma. Superfatted soaps might pass the virility test.

If the skin is exceedingly dry, however, don't use soap and water in the morning. Or in the evening. Or any time other than when the face is very dirty and the extra power of pure soap is mandatory. Rinsable cleansers are all that should be used otherwise, on the condition that moisturizing follows. If hung-up about going the cleanser/moisturizer route, the man may be nearly beyond help. Still, superfatted or cream or other mild soaps are better than the usual variety.

When all's said and done, if a man stubbornly rejects all moisturizing aids, it's his own skin.

Scrubs: Some dermatologists smugly recommend abrasive scrubs for men with dry skin, but such advice is of questionable merit. Dry skin tends to be thinner than other types to begin with. The pores are seldom, if ever, enlarged. This skin may have a web of superficial lines around the eyes and mouth. Rough it up more? Logically, scrubs should be avoided like the plague by any man with dry skin.

Astringents: They are more drying than soap. They would serve no other purpose than to rob more sorely needed moisture from the skin.

Moisturizing: It should now be abundantly clear that moisturizing is the key to helping offset dry skin. Water must first be replaced, otherwise the barrier against evaporation has very little, if any, moisture to entrap. How to replace it? That neat and nifty performing-seal routine. *Splash.* Then spread the moisturizer on the damp face. Men with dry skin can use creamier moisturizers if they choose, but they should double-check in the mirror to be certain an unattractive visible film doesn't show after air drying the face. Throughout the day dousing the face with a little water and "palming" it dry is a good idea.

TWO-FACED
COMBINATION SKIN

It's not unusual for a man, as a consequence of shaving, to have combination skin, say oily at the so-called T-zone (across the forehead and down the nose) but normal or even dry on the cheeks and bearded areas. For inexplicable reasons, patches of dry skin may reside on an otherwise normal or even oily skin. Boring, no doubt, and time-consuming too, but these combination skins must be treated area by area according to each particular skin type.

TOUCHY
SENSITIVE SKIN

Although sensitive skin is usually associated with dry skin, some men's skin will exhibit the characteristics of other skin types and still be unusually irritated by soap, aftershaves, or any number of products. Often rather reddish, though not automatically because of burst capillaries or thinness, sensitive skin presents big problems. Even water can sting. Shaving may be unbearable. Probably the skin has been abused over an extended period of time. If using rinsable cleansers and moisturizers with no fragrance doesn't improve the skin's sensitivity, the need to seek medical aid is inevitable.

CHAPTER **11**
BLEMISHED REPUTATION
COMPLEXION PROBLEMS

Time was when the only consolation for the guy with acne was to describe himself rakishly as the horniest fellow in town. While it's true that blackheads and pimples may indicate overly activating hormones, sexual activity or the lack thereof, even self-styled, cannot cause, aggravate, alleviate, or cure complexion woes. Sex as therapy is fine for the mind but not for the face.

PLUGGED UP
WHITEHEADS, BLACKHEADS

Fundamentally, if a man could keep his pores consistently unclogged, his face would be well on the way to being free of complexion worries. Contrary to old wives' tales, skin eruptions are usually not the result of dirtiness, although perhaps they are heightened by uncleanliness. What's happening beneath the skin's surface is more telling about what's seen above.

For reasons not always explainable, the pores (or ducts) of the skin become plugged with sebum (that oily-waxy secretion of the sebaceous glands—See Chapter 10), which consequently can't complete its journey to the skin's surface. But oil production continues, increasing the amount of trapped sebum. At first the "plug" is fairly colorless. At this point it's commonly called a whitehead. After some time, however, the "plug" oxidizes and turns even darker with

the presence of the skin-protecting pigment melanin. Now the whitehead has been transformed into the classic blackhead.

Still the sebum production continues without any external exit. Enzyme action splits the oils into irritating acids. An inflammation (soreness, redness) results. Eventually something's got to give, usually the follicle walls themselves. They rupture, releasing the acids, oils, bacteria, and sebum into surrounding tissues without a welcome mat, producing more inflammation. The body fights back by increasing the number of white blood cells, which in turn create pus, which results in a pimple, also called a pustule. Ugh.

As should now be evident, blackheads and pimples are ironically produced by the same mechanism that under different circumstances normally protects the

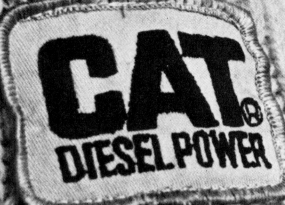

skin's surface by creating the acid mantle. Excessive sebum production, which nearly always occurs during puberty, disrupts the skin's proper functioning.

Even men past adolescence with otherwise flawless complexions sprout an occasional blackhead. It's inevitable. Of course, a blackhead needn't necessarily turn into a pimple (which is a low-grade infection), but if clogging persists, and in great numbers, expect no good to come.

Since blackheads and pimples are not necessarily caused by dirt but by the pores clogging under the skin instead, *special* soaps or scrubs are of little help. Why, then, is such importance granted to cleansing? Because frequent facial washing helps to reduce some plug formations and simultaneously helps eliminate some of the skin's oiliness, both of which can aggravate the situation. Astringents, too, offer assistance.

One way to prevent blackheads culminating inexorably into pimples is to get rid of them before they have the chance. Nearly everyone says that blackheads should only be removed by skin specialists, either dermatologists or facialists, since improper extraction can lead to a spreading infection. In theory, this is absolutely true. In practice, what man can afford the time and expense to undergo a professional facial or to call a dermatologist every time an isolated blackhead or two pops up? These should be removed as quickly as possible before they complete their nasty journey.

If a man doesn't know the correct way to manually squeeze a blackhead (impossible to describe verbally), then he shouldn't attempt it. But the next time he visits a doctor, he can ask to be shown.

The medical term for a blackhead is comedo. Some comedo extractors, fairly simple to operate, are sold in drugstores. One end of the extractor is pointed in order to puncture and loosen the plug. The spoonlike other end has a small round hole to center over the blackhead. When pressure is applied downward, the plug should be forced up and out. Unfortunately, if the entire plug is not removed or if the squeezing is too rough, the skin can be irritated, and infection may follow. Extractors must be scrupulously clean and should be disinfected prior to and after every use. Before extracting a blackhead, the plug should first be softened as much as possible with warm-water compresses (saturated cotton or gauze pads) for three or four minutes. Naturally, the skin should also be dis-

infected after extraction. A cotton ball saturated in alcohol may sting but will reduce the risk of complications.

About pimples. *Never* squeeze them. Repeat, *never*. You can infect yourself. One dermatologist calls the triangular area from the top point between the eyebrows and the lower points at the corners of the mouth "the triangle of death" to terrorize pimple-squeezers into desisting. If not yourself, you can bump off your skin by self-administration. Trust cleanliness and time. And in the future, keep your pores unblocked.

THE PITS
ACNE

Uncontrolled blackheads and pimples can lead to acne. Usually considered an adolescent problem, acne is not uncommon in adults. Several types exist, and medical attention is always recommended.

As in the case of blackheads, hormonal secretions activate increased oil production within the sebaceous glands, enlarging them. While most of the oils reach the skin's surface, some oils are clogged beneath as fatty-waxy plugs. When the damned dammed plugs burst, pimples and even boillike lesions appear. If the body's antibodies can't subjugate the internal infection, it spreads. Disfigurement from acne may be lifelong.

Acne is incurable. However, it is controllable. Unfortunately, too many myths surround it. Diet does *not* affect it; rest does *not* eliminate it; sex does *not* reduce it; antibacterial soaps do *not* affect the primary cause, but do help retard spreading of secondary infection; the sun *does* help.

Since acne's disruptive activity takes place beneath the skin, what's done on the surface topically is usually inefficient.

One independent study concludes that only four medications found in over-the-counter remedies are considered effective by most dermatologists in treating acne. These are benzoyl peroxide, sulfur, resorcinol, and salicylic acid. Each to some degree inflames the skin and causes it to peel. The strongest is benzoyl peroxide.

Since nonprescription medications are required to

list ingredients on their labels, a man with acne should avoid products that contain none of the above-named components. However, there's another consideration. Among the milder formulas, combinations of sulfur (2 to 10 percent) with at least 2 percent resorcinol or salicylic acid must be maintained if the remedy is to be effective. Unfortunately, many labels don't list the percentages of ingredients.

The message is clear, even if the face isn't: Little heed should be given to exorbitant claims. The ingredients listed on the label are what count. Ignore words like "antibacterial." Although bacteria are the sources of enzymes, which break down the oils, they can't be reached by antibacterial agents applied to the skin's surface. Plain old soap will do as much as products lacking the proven medications.

Some people believe only dermatologists should be consulted about continual skin eruptions. Not necessarily. Since one form of treatment is relatively simple—oral antibiotics may check the infection—a family doctor can handle the situation. If he can't, he'll recommend someone who can.

While the sun is usually the vilest villain against the skin, it's a hero for blemish sufferers. Ultraviolet rays are a natural blackhead and pimple retardant, since they dry up the excess oils. Sun lamps theoretically work as well, but there's always the built-in danger of overexposure and facial burning. Even the sun itself must be taken in moderation, and without greasy lotions or oils.

HEARTBREAK
ECZEMA, PSORIASIS

Both these diseases—and *diseases* they are—are characterized by persistently itchy, reddened skin. Like many skin complaints, they cannot presently be cured, but they can be controlled, although almost never by self-prescription. Eczema and psoriasis are mostly mysteries. In psoriasis, the creeping scaliness and the watery liquid that may exude when the scales are scraped away may suggest a malformation in the cellular structure of the epidermis. Such may or may not be the case with eczema. Some over-the-counter "remedies" can benumb the itchiness, but consulting a physician or dermatologist is imperative if any improvement in the skin is hoped for. When specially prescribed measures have checked the primary manifestations of the diseases, then the doctor will usually prescribe simple lotions or creams to keep the problem under wraps. However, if these are discontinued from a false sense of well-being, the disease will reawaken with the same force as before. Medical assistance will then again be necessary before the situation can be ameliorated sufficiently to allow for easier control.

CHAPTER 12

MORNING MALE
SHAVING

Dismissing the obvious drawbacks, the *castrati* of the Middle Ages had two advantages over ordinary men: Their operatic voices were sublime, if high-pitched; and they never had to shave. Short of such extreme countermeasures, most men face the daily drudge of shaving. Much influenced by sex hormones, prepuberty's peach fuzz becomes coarse stubble with the coming of age. Contrary to myth, shaving doesn't make the beard grow faster or denser or tougher. Shaved whiskers are only more inflexible, thus seeming stronger. The beard does coarsen in later years as a perverse compensation for hair loss atop the head. If you opt for facial hair, however, be sure to consult Chapter 8, "Fringe Benefits: Facial Hair."

EDGE WISE
SHAVING METHODS

Although it's generally conceded that a razor blade yields a smoother, closer shave than an electric shaver, many variables come into play. Yet, the preoccupation with receiving a *close* shave can become a mania. A smarter goal is obtaining a *mild* shave, one that doesn't irritate the skin. If the shave happens to be close, that's a happy bonus.

Reputedly electric shavers are gentler to the face than razor blades, but little scientific research supports this claim. When all is said and done, the choice of shaving method—the wet (blade) system versus the dry (electric shaver) technique—depends upon individual preference and experience. Quick touch-ups are less time-consuming with an electric shaver. But treating shaving like a morning marathon is stupid. Most men don't know the right way to shave: They hurry and they hack. Shaving's prologue and epilogue are as important as whether the shave is wet or dry.

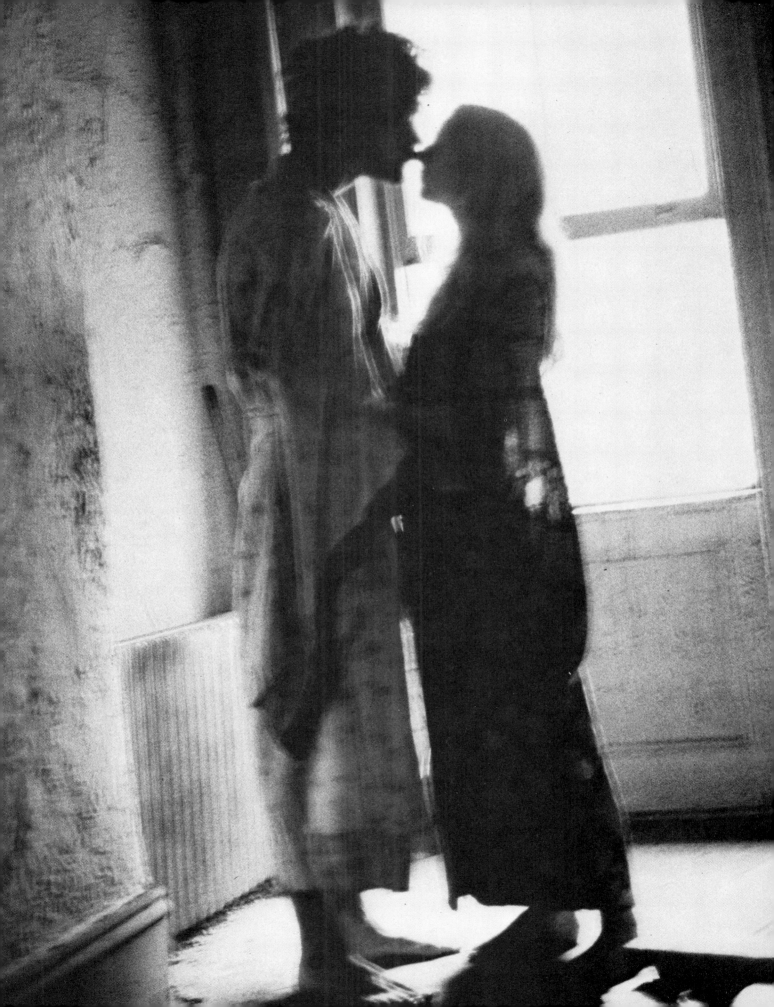

The Prologue

Whichever system is used, a man must prepare his face for the onslaught of shaving. But since wet and dry shaving work on opposing principles, the preliminaries differ. Both should begin with a thorough cleansing of the face to remove any oils from the beard that could detract from the efficiency of the cutting edge or edges.

Blade Shaving: Although most fellows think shaving creams help them receive the closest possible shaves, they're wrong. Sudsing profusely with soap and water, rinsing the face, then swiping with the razor will remove more stubble . . . and more epidermis . . . and hurt like hell.

Shaving preparations were developed for two primary reasons: (1) to wet the beard; and (2) to lubricate the skin. Shaving discomfort and safety depend upon both of these actions. Discomfort arises when the beard resists the blade (insufficient wetting to soften the beard) and when the friction of the razor scrapes against the skin (failure to lubricate the face for easier razor glide). A third function of shaving creams is to swell the beard to make it stand upright so that the whiskers offer bigger, plumper, softer targets.

Just as moisturizers, strictly speaking, can't moisturize the skin but can only entrap hand-fed water within it, similarly, shaving creams or foams alone can't wet the beard. However, these preparations can accelerate the wetting and hold water that has been abundantly splashed onto the whiskers. Moisture is central to a good blade shave, since it reduces beard strength by about 60 percent. Good ol' water, then, again proves its worth as a face-saver. Before putting on a shaving preparation, you should splash the face and neck with hot water for a minimum of one full minute; two is better. (A lengthy washing with soap and water prior to this splashing starts the wetting and softening process.)

Shaving preparations are classified as foam and nonfoam types. The most widely used nonfoam preparation is the typical brushless shaving cream that is applied directly to the wet face from the tube. As the name signifies, this variety doesn't foam. Nor does it barricade moisture within the beard as effectively as foam products, which contain more water in their formulations. Extra time and care must be taken to prewet and presoften the beard. But brushless creams compensate for their inferior wetting with superior lubrication, reducing the risk of razor burn. Their lower alkalinity makes them less oil-robbing for men with dry, flaking, or sensitive skin.

Aerosol creams are favored by most men among the foaming shaving preparations. Foam densities, wetting, and lubricating vary from brand to brand. Thin, watery foams offer minimal lubrication.

The main ingredients in shaving foams are soap and water plus assorted goodies to lubricate, disinfect, and protect. The high alkalinity softens beards more than brushless creams and also removes more oil. Men with greasy skin are best served with foaming preparations.

Widely used menthol doesn't dramatically affect the shave but does impart a cooling sensation. Fragrances are added only for psychological value. Since preparations should be totally rinsed away after shaving, leftover fragrance is not very concentrated. The term *medicated* refers to germicides and healing ingredients usually found in conventional foams in smaller but usually acceptable proportions.

Borrowing from the mystique of the fast-disappearing barber shave, some manufacturers suggest that heat is today's missing ingredient. Enter hot lathers either in cans or via dispensers that attach to cans. The theory is that heat causes the beard to be receptive to moisture (true) and increases foam efficiency (debatable).

Certain shaving foam makers refuse to endorse hot-lather concepts, claiming that only the exterior of the molecules is heated, bursting to cool during the shave. Others say too much heat can imbalance careful formulations. While still others suggest that if hot lather feels good, that's what counts. The potential risk of hot lathers is that a man might cut down on his prewetting time, supposing the hot lather will do all the work. It won't.

Once a shaving preparation is applied, the water in the formula continues wetting the beard while depositing a filmy protection to promote razor glide. For these reasons, the product is enhanced if the beard is soaked with the foam for two minutes before wielding the blade. Adapting this truth, certain companies have introduced preshave emulsions that are spread on the face to remain there for a minute before adding a regular foam, waiting another minute, and then shaving.

For the fellow with tender skin, the two-step application of shaving preparations optimizes lubricity.

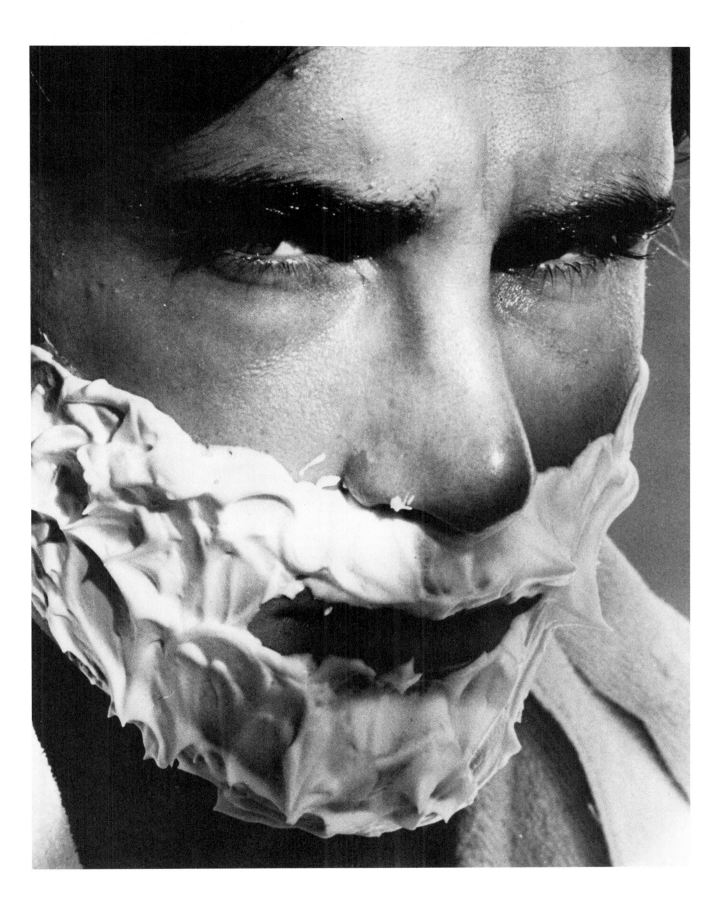

Trying to formulate the same degree of protection in a one-step foam would be impossible without reducing the foam's ability to wet the beard. However, specialized preshave formulations aren't the only means to augment lubrication. Any moisturizer spread onto the wet face before the foam is applied is an excellent alternative.

Electric Shaving: In contrast to wet shaving, when the beard should be as wet and soft as possible, electric shavers operate best against dry and hard beards. Why? Because softened whiskers can evasively bend away from the implement without penetrating the foils on the shaver's head. Since the clipping takes place under these foils, the beard must be stiff, and the stiffest whiskers are the driest whiskers. Individual beard hairs must be hard enough to stand alone. When so united, they're ready to fall.

Oils both soften the beard and help the whiskers elude the cutting edges of the electric shaver. A thorough cleansing with soap and water or a rinsable cleanser de-oils the face and beard. Yet the beard is simultaneously slightly softened in the process, while the unlubricated skin remains vulnerable to the friction of the shaver dragging over the face. Enter pre-electric-shaving preparations.

These items should be formulated with enough astringency to stiffen the beard while evaporating quickly, leaving no liquid behind. At the same time, the preparations should deposit enough coating to the skin so the shaver can glide over the face without skimming. Unfortunately, these two actions can be mutually exclusive unless the preparations are created with great finesse. Not all those sold are.

The Center Stages

After preparing the face for shaving, many men are careless during dewhiskering. Although severe cuts are likelier with a blade, any face can be nicked and gouged with an electric shaver relentlessly ground into the skin. Even when extreme care is taken, micro-abrasions are inevitable. While soothing them takes place during the epilogue (see page 92), certain shaving techniques invite irritations and should therefore be avoided.

Probably the most destructive way to direct either blade or shaver is against the beard's grain. Shaving this way does produce closer results, but it can also result in whiskers being clipped off beneath the sur-

face of the skin. Acting like foreign objects, the sharp ends of the beard hairs now jab at the surrounding tissues. And the body responds as it would if an alien particle were introduced beneath the skin: Inflammation, possibly infection, ensues. This reaction, to which men with curly and coarse beards are more susceptible, is the same as the development of ingrown hairs, which can occur either when the hair shaft fails to exit from the pore but pushes into the tissues surrounding the hair follicle, or when the hair shaft, after exiting the pore opening, curves back and lodges its sharp head into the skin, growing inward. Either way, the consequence is painful, and infection may ensue. The guilty head of the hair should be *gently* extracted with tweezers and the skin treated with a disinfectant.

To repeat, the quest for the closest possible shave is usually a rash decision.

Blade Shaving: A dull razor blade can undo all the good of proper facial preparation. Old cutting edges traumatize the skin by pulling against the beard. The resulting ragged stubble is more likely to be caught in the skin, threatening the development of ingrown hairs, especially on the tender neck area. A tiny layer of skin is always removed during shaving, but when the blades are dull, the skin will look scratchy and blotchy. Changing blades may cost more, but fresh blades are less costly to the face's appearance. How frequently blades must be changed will depend upon beard strength, the quality of the blades themselves, and how often you shave. Allowing more than a week to pass without inserting a new blade is risky. Blades should never be wiped with tissues or towels, since such action dulls them faster.

For a healthy shave, the sharp razor blade should also be antiseptically clean and residue-free. First rinse it under a rush of water. Now pour a little alcohol (or mouthwash or aftershave lotion) over the blade to remove bacteria. Rinse again. (Repeat at the shave's conclusion.) Some may find these steps overly conscientious. Perhaps. But they can't hurt and might help. Infections from blade shaving are not prevalent, even likely, but why take chances? Keeping the face as bacteria-free as possible also helps control unsightly blemishes.

Even during shaving, reliable water is especially beneficial. Wetting the blade with hot water before the first swath and throughout the shave makes the entire operation easier. Rinsing the shaved hairs from

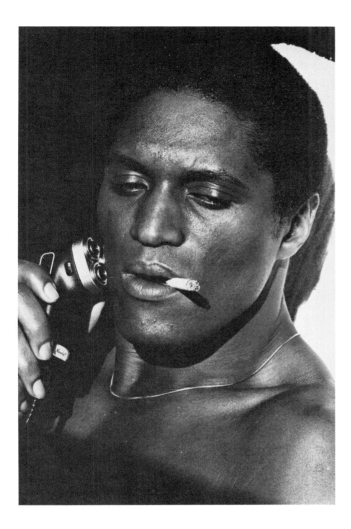 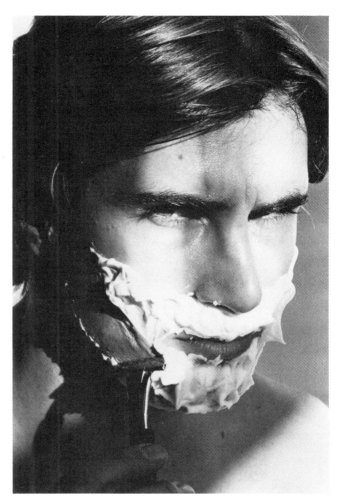

the razor's edge eliminates possible deflections and irritants.

Since the chin and upper lip have the heaviest concentration of coarse beard hairs, leaving these two zones to the last is best, so that they can be softened to the maximum by the water and foam.

As mentioned, shaving foams contain alkaline soap, which is drying to the skin. Therefore, just as you rinse thoroughly after washing the face, so you should splash, splash, splash with warm water after shaving to make certain every trace of foam is removed. Failure to do so leaves a foreign residue on the face which invites irritation.

Electric Shaving: Trying for too close a shave with an electric shaver is as destructive to the skin as overshaving with a blade. A gentle shave is always preferable to a dangerously close one, even if shaving must be done twice daily.

Although electric shavers come in a variety of shapes, they all operate on the same principle; that is, beard hairs penetrating the perforations of the metal head are shorn by moving blades on the other side of the foil or disks. By constantly shaving and reshaving the beard in circular motions, a man not only goes against the beard's grain, but he also is probably producing differing lengths of the stubble, which may be ragged. The results? A greater propensity toward ingrown hairs and nicks and irritations. Methodical, gentle shaving makes more sense. Never overdo.

Unfortunately, some pre-electric-shaving preparations leave a stubbornly oily-greasy residue on the face. Sometimes it can be removed by dousing with an aftershave lotion and rinsing. More tenacious types may require strong astringents or full-strength alcohol to be rid of their presence. Thus, any benefits (real or imagined) from electric shaving to dry-skinned individuals may be blown if drying astringents or alcohol must be rubbed on the face to offset the undesirable consequences of an undesirable pre-electric-shaving preparation.

To operate at best efficiency, the cutting edges of electric shavers should be sharp and scrupulously clean. That means cleaning them following every shave. But *never* blow the surfaces clean. The minute beard clippings might lodge themselves in your eyes, both a painful and a hazardous event. Those dumb-looking brushes that manufacturers supply are the only smart way to keep the shavers clean. Follow directions.

When the cutting edges become dull—your skin will tell you—replace them.

The Epilogue

With the dewhiskering completed, the residual shaving preparation thoroughly removed from the face, and the shaving implement cleaned, is the shave concluded? No way, for either the dry or the wet system.

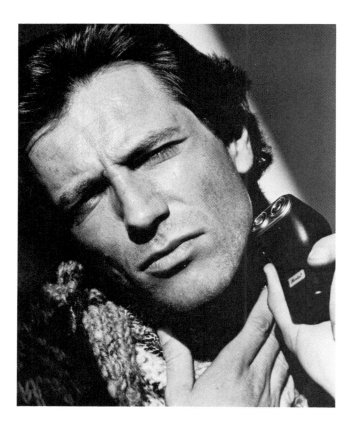

Though you tried your best to be gentle, the skin has been abraded. Parts of it may be nearly raw. Vulnerable to bacterial attack, your face needs protection and soothing.

Unless the face is exceptionally dry or sensitive, disinfecting it with a splash of aftershave lotion is a precaution that can't hurt but might sting. Witch hazel smarts less but doesn't include the lubricants and agents usually found in aftershaves. Colognes sting more, with less benefits. Alcohols or astringents may be used by men with oily skin, but they'll also be face slapping. An aftershave balm is more soothing while it disinfects.

Now you're finished, right? Wrong. Remember, moisturizing the face is essential even for oily skin. Almost immediately after dousing on the aftershave lotion (or alcohol or witch hazel or astringent), splash away the potentially drying agents by cupping heaping handfuls of lukewarm water over the face for a minute or more. Palm away the excess water. Apply a thin film of aftershaving balm over the face and neck to seal in the moisture. (Or skip the potentially drying agents altogether, splash like crazy after shaving, then apply the balm for a one-step antiseptic and soother.) In place of the aftershave balm, any moisturizer is acceptable but probably won't have any of the healing agents (unless it is specifically designated an aftershave *moisturizer*) with which lotions or balms are formulated.

ROUGH GOING
SHAVING PROBLEMS

If these shaving procedures are followed for either blade or shaver, discomfort and irritation should be minimal. Abnormal sensitivity indicates consulting a dermatologist.

However, some males—especially black men—are consistently subjected to the touchy problem of ingrown hairs. These can be aggravated to the point of scarring. Even when these fellows don't shave too close or against the grain, the inborn tendency of the beard to curve into the skin commonly produces "bumps." Experimenting with both shaving systems, they may find that neither reduces the dilemma. In such instances, depilatories (complete with all their risks) can be explored. Unfortunately, since depilator-

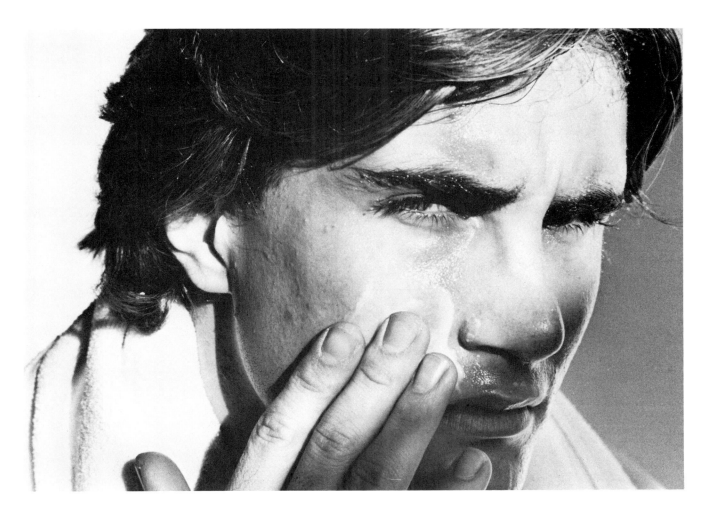

ies are chemical agents to destroy hair, they're not exactly the kindest way to treat your skin, which must also come in contact with the harsh creams.

Before using a depilatory, a man should first test for unusual skin sensitivity by applying the product to a *small* portion of the beard for the maximum time specified on the label, then removing it according to instructions and waiting for twenty-four hours. If any rash or discomfort occurs, forget about that brand of depilatory.

The drawback of depilatories is that many men experience rashes as a result of using them. In some cases these can be offset by applying warm-water compresses to the skin for several minutes after removing the whiskers, cleansing the face thoroughly, rinsing again, then soothing the face with a moisturizing cream. (For more detailed information about using depilatories to remove unwanted body hair, see page 150.)

For certain individuals, the only way to overcome the rough goings of shaving may be to grow a beard (see Chapter 8), but during the initial stages, great care must be taken to guard against ingrowing hairs. However, these should not be plucked; as noted, the tip should be carefully pulled away with tweezers to keep it from lodging its point into the skin. Magnifying mirrors help. And remember to disinfect.

Men with severe acne may also be forced into sprouting facial hair. But shaving can be somewhat beneficial to this kind of skin problem provided the heads of the pustules (pimples) aren't cut and the infection doesn't spread on the skin's surface. Shaving daily with a new blade is highly recommended if the man's personal experience proves wet shaving is easier for him. He should finalize his shave by applying an astringent antiseptic lotion. Using a moisturizer is not recommended for someone with acne or severe blemishes.

CHAPTER **13**

MASQUE FORCE
FACIALS

Once the private domain of pampered society matrons, skin care salons have opened wide their doors to men in recent years. In fact, shops devoted exclusively to men are not uncommon. Although some establishments overplay their services into an esoteric mystique, what they are really promoting is clean skin and protection from damaging products. The fundamental tool of the trade is the facial—cleansing, plus extra nifties like relaxing massage and blemish extraction.

THE SKIN GAME
PROFESSIONAL FACIALS

There's no such thing as a typical professional facial, since nearly every salon claims a secret approach. Of course, such mysteries aren't divulged in detail, otherwise they wouldn't be secrets. Certain masques (various creams or pastes applied to the face to remain there for several minutes or more, reputedly to "nourish" the skin and aid in cleansing) are formulated from Dead Sea mud; *toniques* may be concocted from *herbes de Provence*; creams may be fortified with placenta or perhaps papaya. Besides the exotic ingredients in their products, many skin salons also employ exotic terminology. One skin care center in Manhattan, for example, classifies skin in *twenty* types. The mind swims.

Although methods and methodologies vary from salon to salon, a professional facial will probably incorporate most of the following generalized steps, though not necessarily in this chronology. Some salons won't use any machines other than vaporizers (steamers), so mechanical steps might be performed differently by hand.

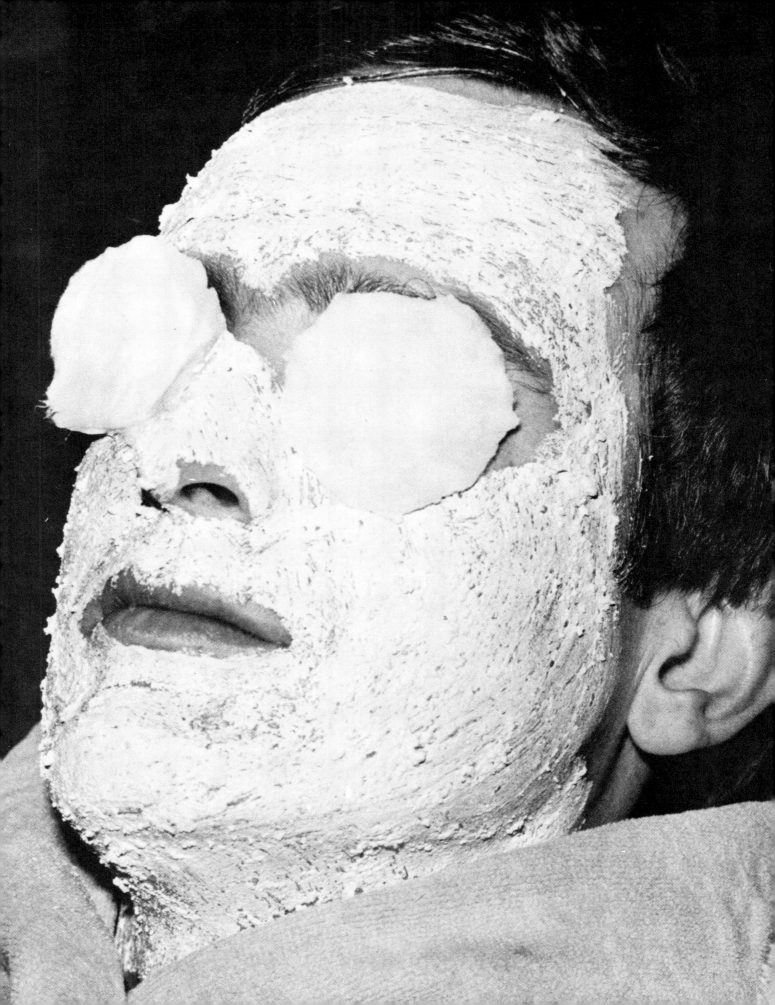

1

First, the skin is analyzed. You're seated before a two-way mirror that magnifies your face. (Some establishments will superficially cleanse the face first.) Ostensibly the two-way magnifier assists the facialist in investigating your skin and determining what, if any, problems you have. Actually, an expert could probably tell without this enlarged scrutiny. You discover in your reflection that your pores look like caverns and pimples resemble inflamed mountains. You realize you need help! This isn't really a tricky fraud. It's just that you see what no one else does unless your friends carry magnifying glasses. Still, since few of us ever really examine our skins carefully, shock treatment can carry home the message that attention must be paid. If your facialist doesn't use a two-way magnifier, mentally congratulate him or her for good taste.

2

After your skin has been analyzed, you may be shown into a private room (if you're not already there), where you're presented with a robe and a contoured reclining chair. Perhaps the lighting is dim and the music is soft. You lie back. Then the mist, machine-produced from a vaporizer, may descend. It films your face with moist drops and reputedly opens the pores. (In some salons, you'll lower your face—with a towel as a hood—over a brew of herbs to be steamed into your skin.)

3

Some salons withhold the steaming until later. In that case, your face will first be massaged with an appropriate cream to cleanse it. Blood circulation is stimulated. The cream is probably removed with cotton.

4

Another cleansing follows. It may be performed with a soft, automated brush that is meant to whirl away surface dirt and dead cells. A mild electrical shock may or may not be induced by another machine, supposedly to soften hardened sebum. A vacuumlike machine sucks away any debris. (Several experts insist that this is more showmanship than efficiency.) If the vaporizer wasn't turned on earlier, it more than likely will be now.

5

The facialist extracts, by hand, any impurities or blemishes.

6

More misty droplets may or may not be directed on your face. In some instances, the skin will be sprayed with extracts or plants for "aroma therapy." The skin is cleansed one more time. This step is usually called deep-pore cleansing. Creams may be spread, followed by a drying or a nondrying masque. (Drying masques are quite universally used on oily skins.)

7

When the masque is removed with the appropriate lotions, you'll hopefully be treated to a massage of the face, neck, and shoulders that will make you want to melt. Relax. Enjoy. Fantasize.

8

Get set. You may be sprayed again. Or maybe not. It depends upon the salon.

9

A light moisturizer or protective cream will usually be applied before you leave your chair of luxury.

10

Your facialist will suggest how you should care for your skin at home. The recommendation will almost inevitably include a regimen based on the salon's proprietary products.

11

You settle your tab, leave a tip, and face the world with a glowing face.

That's right, you'll have on a healthy glow. That glow is what convinces many men that facials must do wonders for their skin. Well, wonders cease. The glow is the manifestation of the masque effect, a natural phenomenon that occurs after skin is manipulated. This extensive massage, combined with aromatic products, causes the inner blood vessels to expand, plumping the skin and making its tone look more youthfully pinkish. But the masque effect is short-lived, this visible "improvement" only temporary. Many medical men say that facials primarily plump up a man's ego (in direct proportion to the masque effect) but do little for the skin's health.

It's essentially true that what you pay for when you're given a facial is a clean face. Plus the relaxation. And the relaxation aspect should not be pooh-poohed. Stress is skin ravaging. Unless someone is allergic to the products or unless the facialist is inept, certainly no evidence exists that facials are harmful. To the contrary, many men avidly endorse them, insisting that they've seen remarkable improvements in their skin over a period of time from facials.

The most difficult aspect to evaluate about professional facials is their practitioners' claims that these prevent potential skin problems, especially premature aging. As mentioned earlier, preventive measures can only be followed on faith. That very faith may help prevent the negative happenings. Who can say? As one prominent dermatologist has said, "I will not blanketly condemn facials. Truthfully, I don't know if they help the skin or not. People who have facials generally do everything they can to enhance their skin's appearance, so they usually have more attractive skin. How much facials have to do with it, I have no way of gauging."

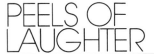

PEELS OF LAUGHTER
AT-HOME FACIALS

Egg masques, tube masques, masque scrubs, and do-it-yourself varieties *probably* offer less hope for *long-range* benefits than do professional facials. But note the "probably" and the "long-range."

Some masques-in-a-tube sold by prestige groomers are promoted for their deep cleansing. Hogwash. As seen during professional facials, at least one or two cleansings always precede masque application. Obviously masques alone aren't the most effective cleansers.

Other companies more honestly say that their face masques tone up the skin temporarily, that they are offered "to break the five o'clock doldrums." The tightening action of the masque does create a temporarily tingling masque effect.

One possibly beneficial side effect of at-home facials is the removal of dead cells from the skin's surface. Of course, scrubbing with a rough sponge will do the same.

At-home facials are either of the rinse-off or peel-off kind. Not surprisingly, the rinse-off ones are removed with water, while the peel-off types do just that. Depending upon their ingredients, one is neither superior nor inferior to the other. Peel-off masques, however, don't always peel cleanly away, so a fellow may need to spend extra time riding his face of sticky little nurdles.

Masques can be amusing. They can also be relaxing. But they can't replace conscientious cleansing and protecting. If you want to indulge, go ahead. At-home facials shouldn't hurt unless you have very sensitive skin. Accept masques for what they are. A few belts of booze create a short-term glow too. But dry martinis don't qualify as skin care products.

CHAPTER 14

BORDER LINES

FIGHTING WRINKLES

Who said wrinkles give a man's face character? Probably someone descended from a prune. True, an unlined face on an adult male looks eerily unreal. But, as these names indicate, "turkey neck," "squirrel jowls," "crow's feet," and the like are hardly sought-after compliments. Wrinkles are correctly associated with age, since time eventually leaves its marks. But premature wrinkling needn't be accepted blithely. While it's true that the only sure way to rejuvenate a wrinkled face is via cosmetic surgery (see Chapter 17), why not consider a few preventive measures?

X-RATED RAYS
ENVIRONMENTAL FACTORS

There's little good in a deep suntan other than the way it looks. Since tanning is one way the skin protects itself from the sun's harmful rays, a healthy tan isn't really healthy at all, beyond the psychological lift of seeing it in a mirror. In fact, too much exposure to the sun is downright hazardous to the skin.

Without going into the biological aspects, suffice it to say that the destructive effects of the sun are cumulative and at some point irreversible. In addition to increasing the possibility of skin cancer, the sun's burning rays attack the tissues at the base of the skin.

These tissues support the skin and give it its elasticity. When they are damaged or destroyed, the skin "collapses"; wrinkling ensues. These tissues do not regenerate themselves. Once real wrinkles are formed (as opposed to superficial wrinkles, or lines on the surface of the face accompanying dry skin), they're with you for life unless they're artificially removed.

But, then, you already know that too much sun is bad for the skin, don't you? Remember the fact, too, the next time you're basking on a beach: Those tanning rays are mapping out your face's future.

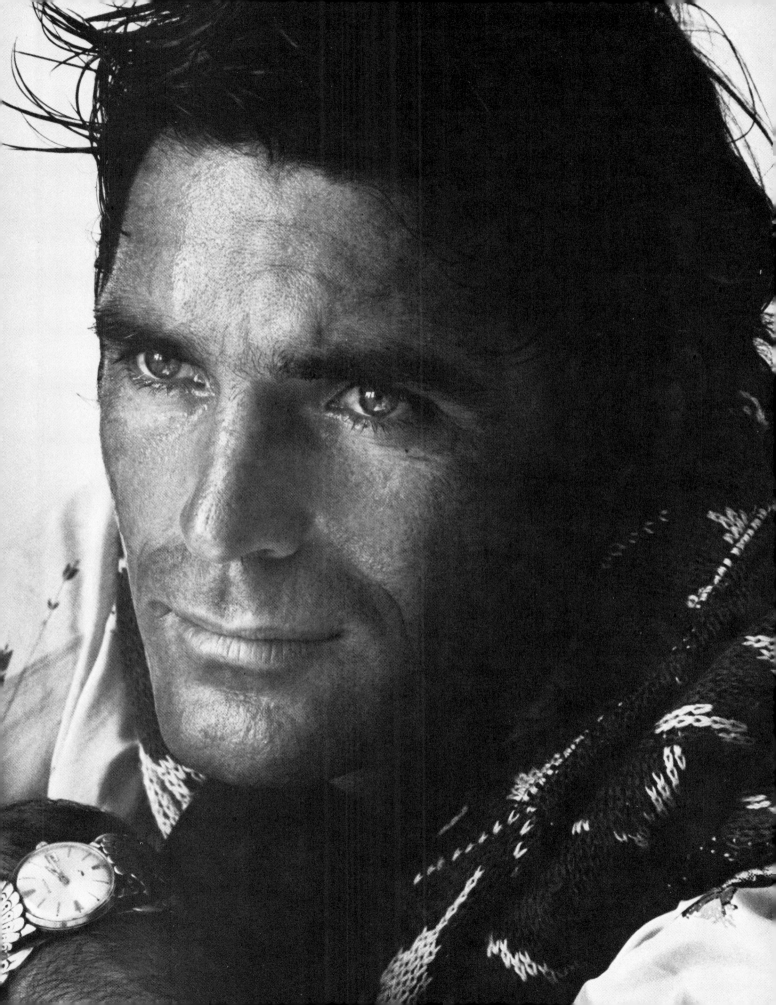

WATERING HOLES
MOISTURIZING FACTORS

You also already know that the skin needs moisture to look and stay young. Splashing water on the face and entrapping it there with a moisturizing film is the best way to keep the face moistly protected. When the skin hasn't sufficient moisture, superficial lines appear. These may not be *real* wrinkles...yet. Without therapeutic water, the lines become more pronounced. Eventually, when the face becomes dehydrated, the supporting tissues can't do their job.

As often as the fact has been driven home, it bears another repetition: Accelerated wrinkling occurs without proper moisturization. You can't stop wrinkles entirely, but you'll never slow them down if you follow the course of top-speed neglect.

CREAMED
COSMETIC FACTORS

Numerous antiwrinkle creams are sold. Other than temporarily plumping up the skin, these creams don't truly *remove* wrinkles; they disguise them for a short while. Hydration remains the key. However, some creams may "fluff" the skin by superficially irritating it and causing it to become a bit swollen. It is only a chemical reaction; some wrinkles may appear to be removed. The results of the creams might also give the appearance of a puffy-eyed hangover. Tender skin around the eyes may be overly irritated. Certain methods of applying cosmetics—the standard advice is "up and out"—supposedly retard wrinkling. Nonsense.

INSTANT REPLAY
EXERCISE FACTORS

Do facial exercises help or not? Are you surprised to hear that some people claim that cosmetic surgery might be avoided if you would only contort your features more, while others denounce ear wriggling, eye shutting, eyebrow raising, toothless smiling, and teeth clenching as silly wastes of time? No, you're not surprised.

It's unlikely that anyone will ever know for sure which view is correct, simply because human guinea pigs aren't likely to ever undergo laboratory experiments exercising one side of their faces to the total exclusion of the other half. Theoretically, enlarging a muscle mass should stretch the skin, thereby reducing some wrinkles. But if rigorous exercise only increases biceps slightly, monumental efforts would be required to strengthen forehead muscles to the extent of removing furrows. Besides, who wants a bulging forehead?

Certain facialists claim they can remove wrinkles through massage, a kind of passive exercise for the skin. The masque-effect phenomenon has previously been noted. It illustrates that wrinkles may be *apparently* removed by puffing the skin, but these lines reappear shortly. Small lines (not true wrinkles) may not reappear at all or at least as quickly as established ones if the skin is sufficiently hydrated. To some degree, facial massage quickens the sloughing of accumulated dead cells on the face. A thinned skin may appear slightly less wrinkled over a period of time.

In general, exercise stretches the muscles, making them more supple. A wise goal for the body, but do we really want our facial muscles stretched? Might not that make any wrinkles even more apparent? That's exactly what some physicians say, who suggest that the only method of ridding true wrinkles is through plastic surgery. They also claim that too vigorous manipulation of the face can damage connecting tissues at the base of the skin and cause premature wrinkling.

Some specialists also assert that smiling too much can cause deeper "expression lines." Ever-beaming individuals do appear to possess more deeply etched wrinkles near their lips and at the eyes. But giving up smiling is a very dour alternative.

LIT UP
SMOKING FACTORS

Evidence indicates that face wrinkles, particularly crow's feet (that network of fine lines starting at the

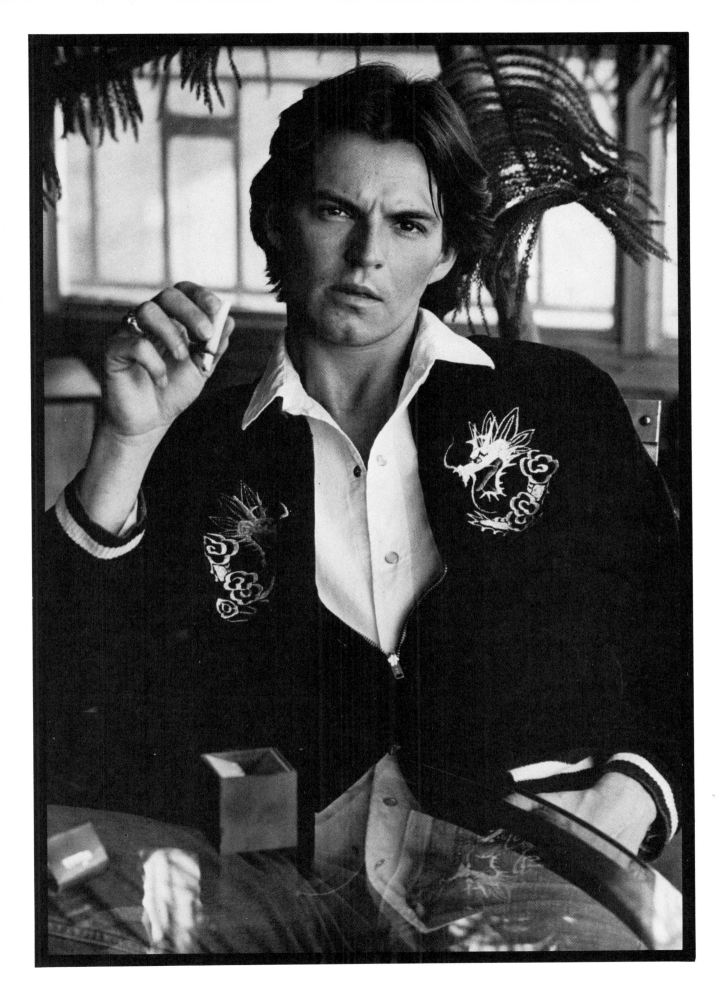

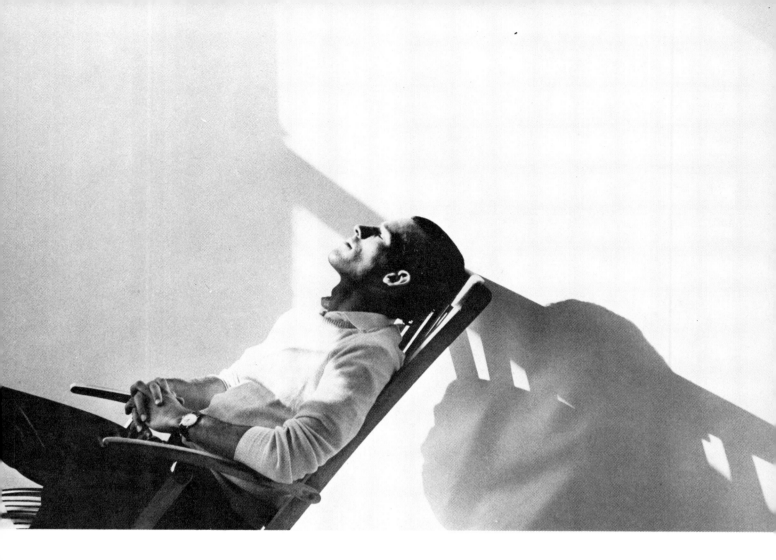

corners of the eyes), are hastened if you smoke. The more you smoke, the deeper these lines can become. Cigarette smoking causes more wrinkling than pipe smoking. The reasons are unclear. One hypothesis is that heavy smokers squint more than nonsmokers do in order to protect their eyes from the smoke. If this is true, the appearance of cigarette-related wrinkles might support the notion that squinting exercises to remove wrinkles (or prevent them) around the eyes could work exactly in the reverse, producing more of them.

Everyone knows that smoking is dangerously unhealthy, so no preaching will be forthcoming here. However, if you must pollute your system, every morning and night splash your closed (but not clenched) eyelids with warm water, lightly blot them with a tissue, then apply some oil or petroleum jelly

sparingly around the eyes for extra protection. A physiological fact is that the eyes are always dryer than the rest of the face; wrinkles are more likely to appear in this area faster.

DREAMBOAT
REST FACTORS

Sleep unravels care, and possibly premature wrinkling. When we're exhausted, our skin looks sallow, our whole system is sluggish. When we're well rested, our blood (which nourishes the skin) circulates more efficiently. The man who dreams about a healthier, wrinkle-free complexion could do far worse than healthily dreaming longer. Although the widespread notion that illness or lack of sleep causes dark circles to appear under our eyes is under attack — the scientific explanation for these bluish circles is veins too close to thin undereye skin — many morning-after experiences prove that if you carouse indiscreetly, you look like hell. How much sleep is required? Who can say? But three hours a night is damn well pushing your luck. As important as sleep is to appearance and body health, its value is even greater for the psyche. No-sleep torture techniques are among the most effective. Self-torture is for sickies.

THAT OLD FEELING
AGING FACTORS

Aging is a natural process, not the end of the world. A normal amount of lines and wrinkling is inevitable, since with age, bodies lose moisture, and skin loses its elasticity. If we don't keep our systems functioning optimally, the debility of age arrives sooner. Wrinkling tendencies may be influenced by heredity, but mainly we inherit bad habits. Applying a fifty-dollars'per-ounce cream when the body isn't in top condition adds up to zero value.

CHAPTER 15
OFF COLOR
ARTIFICE

During various epochs in history, men have indulged in ostentatious facial powders and paints. Since mankind still exists, dabbling with makeup apparently didn't seriously affect either these men's virility or their fertility. Today, males wearing cosmetics that do something "unnatural" to their faces is frowned upon *if others can tell*. Moisturizers, though suspect, are grudgingly accepted (and not by all) only because their benefits to skin health are demonstrable. However, wearing a pigmented foundation, which can function as a moisturizer, raises eyebrows *if people know*. Although "artifice"—to use a less emotionally charged word than makeup—for men is only barely tolerated and never embraced by society at large, some guys refuse to be bullied. Like it or not, increasing numbers of men are currently doing whatever they feel they have to do to look better. If that includes artifice, tough.

KEEPING A GLOW ON
BRONZERS

Even though medical science has proved that overdoses of sun are lethal to the skin, many men literally play with the fire of the sun's rays and risk skin damage for the ego boost of a suntan. Others, probably smarter, get their glow from a tube. Bronzers, which contain harmless dyes to impart a ruddy color to the face, make an office-imprisoned executive look as if he's just returned from a week in the Bahamas — at a fraction of the price and none of the risk.

Although often considered makeup, strictly speaking, bronzers aren't. Being translucent, they don't mask freckles or blemishes the way opaque cosmetics do; they only darken them while shading the rest of the face as well. The products can be applied on any exposed area of the body, but their use is generally confined to the face and neck.

Using a bronzer isn't tricky once you get the hang of careful application, but when overused, you can

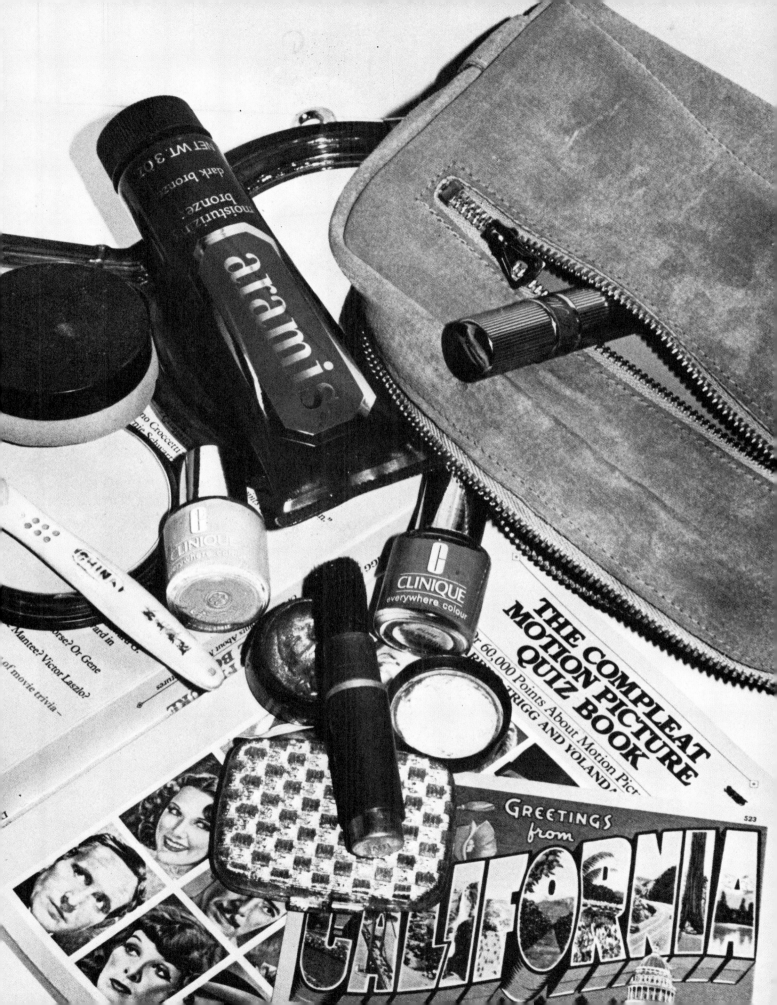

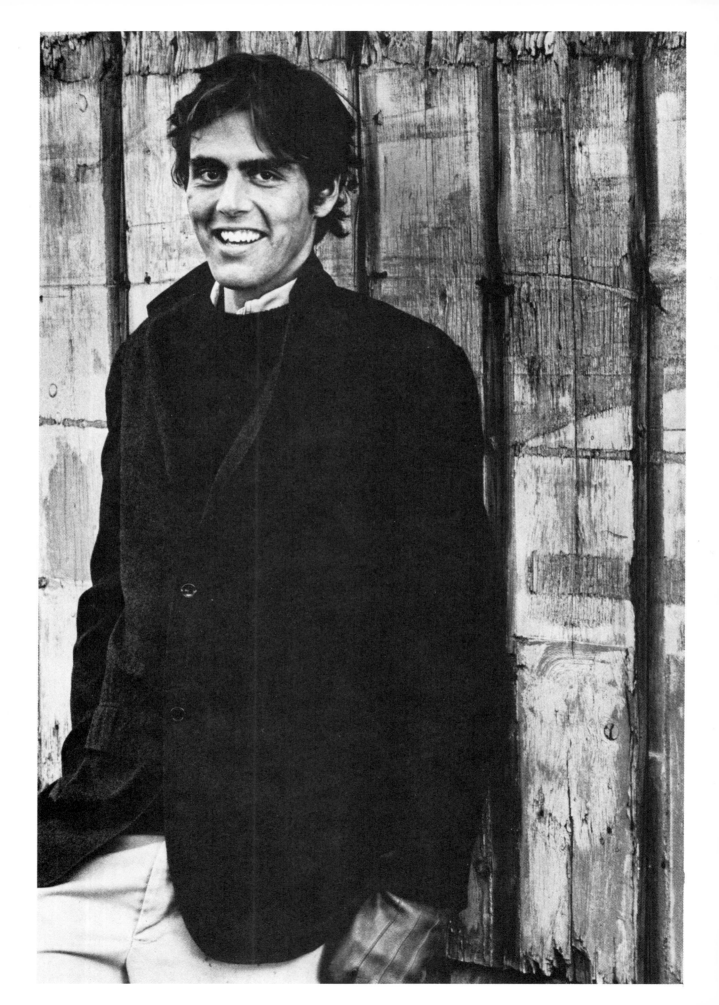

look as if you're wearing latter-day war paint.

Two types of bronzers are available: One form is a gel in a tube; the other, a solid stick variety.

The most popular bronzers today are the gel types. Since they are massaged into the skin with the fingertips, the application technique seems more natural than does that for the stick type. Gels dry faster, which can be advantageous or not.

You can apply bronzing gels using two methods. Either way, working in front of a well-lighted mirror to evaluate the results, always start with scrubbed hands and a clean, freshly shaved face.

The simpler and faster method is to squeeze a small amount of the gel onto your fingertips, rub them together, then quickly spread the bronzer over your face, blending the color evenly onto facial contours and into the hairline. Smooth on small, even dabs of bronzer to highlight the cheeks, forehead, chin, and nose—those areas where natural tans color more deeply.

You can also apply a bronzer by dividing the face into zones: the forehead, the nose, the two cheek areas, and the upper-lip/chin section. Spread the bronzer with the fingertips one area at a time, starting at the forehead and working down. When the entire face is completed, highlight it.

Stick application is easier, though there's a greater natural tendency to overcolor. You simply push the stick *lightly* over the entire face. Some men make the mistake of applying one overall color, failing to consider where natural tanning is lighter (under the chin) or darker (on the cheekbones). Sticks give more opaque coverage if not blended in with the fingertips.

A matter of personal taste: A small amount of talc in a natural shade will tone down either type bronzer and add a matte finish if desired. However, this step may visually cross the borderline into a made-up appearance if subtlety is not applied as well.

Bronzers are formulated to be quick-drying. Don't dawdle. Use little if any, on those areas—the eyelids, the neck immediately beneath the chin, the nostrils, behind the ears—that normally aren't tanned.

Blending into the hair and sideburns is essential to avoid a masklike look. Also, beware the neck area. This is one spot in particular where you must blend carefully, not only for laundry considerations but also to avoid a telltale line of demarcation.

Under casual conditions, water (even light rain) won't streak a bronzer. However, if you perspire ex-cessively, sometimes natural oils will affect the coloration. If so, don't rub your face or neck to remove the perspiration; blot with a tissue instead.

When first using a bronzer, let discretion be your guide. Remember, natural tans build slowly. Start lightly and go deeper in coloration with time.

Hands are usually naturally more pigmented than the face. Unless you're darkening your face considerably, don't apply bronzers to hands. If you do, spread only on the tops, never the palms. Avoid fingers; the wrinkles around knuckles will look dirty, not tanned. Better yet, don't deepen your facial shade so much that you need to worry about your hands.

After applying the bronzer, you should be able to wash away the residue on your palms and fingertips with soap and water. If you've been too slow or have gotten loads of bronzer on your hands, removal may not be easy. Scrubbing with granular hand soap should do the job. But *never* use this type of soap to remove a bronzer from your face.

To remove the stains from the face—and you should always be thorough in removing nightly—wash first with soap and water. Then remove any residue with an astringent soaked in cotton pads. Make extra certain that you've rid all traces from blended areas like the hairline and sideburns. After removing a bronzer, always splash the face with plenty of lukewarm water, palm dry, then moisturize.

Today many bronzers contain moisturizing ingredients. They act as a protective shield against the environment. Some even contain sunscreens (see "Fatherly Sun Advice" in Chapter 27).

So-called moisturizing bronzers should not be applied as you would a moisturizer. Stick to the bronzer steps. However, first treat the face to extra splashes of water, then lightly towel it dry. Bronzers should never be spread on a wet face, lest you obtain uneven results.

Certain companies market only one bronzing shade. The more bronzer applied, the deeper the color. Other firms offer both natural and dark shades. Even so, the amount applied affects color density and depth. Since additional dabs can always be worked into the skin, start sparingly.

Don't douse your face with aftershaves or colognes following bronzing; the alcohol will make the color run. And don't apply a moisturizer over a bronzer. If the bronzer you select isn't a moisturizing one, you can—and should—use a moisturizer under the bronzer, but allow the face to dry first before adding the glow.

Naturally, there's a natural way to bronze: in the good old summer time, that is. It's discussed fully on page 127.

SHADY BUSINESS
MAKEUP

Even when a major cosmetic company finally introduced a makeup kit for men, they didn't have the courage of their conviction. Anticipating some jokes and jibes, the firm called its group of products colouring box for men. Containing no glitter, the kit includes relatively safe eye crayons to conceal circles and highlight lids; a basic black mascara; two pressed powders, with brush, for contouring and shadow-sculpturing the face; a tinted moisturizer that is really a liquid foundation; and a lip gloss.

Other male/mail order companies have been more adventurous. One in Massachusetts, for example, offers powder or water-applied eyecolor for men in midnight green and blue as well as copper brown and shadow gray. (Application of these is discussed later on in this chapter.)

The man who chooses to wear obvious makeup doesn't need forewarning that he may receive some catcalls. Not worrying about subtlety, he can apply the cosmetics (which certainly need not be labled for men) however he chooses. But he should be aware of some of the findings by the American Medical Association about use of cosmetics by women.

"Miracle" Ingredients: There aren't any, only eccentric ones, which are more likely to cause allergic reactions than do the commonplace, time-proved cosmetic ingredients.

Hypoallergenic Products: The term hypoallergenic originally referred to products that were supposed to be "nonallergic." Now it means "least likely" to cause allergies, which doesn't cut much mustard with the one guy in a million who might be allergic to a hypoallergenic soap that millions of others use blissfully and safely. These so-called products offer no insurance that they won't cause allergic reactions among some individuals, only that any ingredients widely known to cause allergies are not included in the formulas. Don't worry what those ingredients are. Why worry? If you have an allergy you should already know what causes it. Don't become a hypochondriac.

Organic Products: No proved superiority or special benefits. Many of the ingredients may not even be natural. If no preservatives are added, these products are more easily contaminated than conventional forms.

Bright Eyed

It's not to everyone's taste, but most out-and-out makeup efforts by the brave (or brazen) men who are into indiscriminate artifice are directed toward their eyes.

Full-fledged eye makeup usually starts with eye shadow. That term is deliberate, since the desired impression is a deeper toned "shadowing" between the eyelid and the eyebrow, particularly from the edge of the eye to the end of the brow, so that it looks as if a shadow has been cast by lavish lashes. Eye shadows come in various forms—crayons, oils, creams, or pressed powders—and are applied either with brushes or fingertips. Generally, though not always, these shadows fall into natural shades of browns and blacks, at least insofar as they are utilized by men.

To "brighten" the shadows, highlighters may also be used. These are lighter toned, such as beige or frosted blue, although some guy could probably discover one in shimmering green. Highlighters, like eye shadows, come in different forms and are either brush- or finger-applied (seldom the latter).

Eyeliners—dark cakes or oils which are applied to the rim of the lids to define eye shape—may or may not be used. Usually in black or brown, eyeliners can be in off-colors. Sometimes they're available in pencils. Types applied with brushes aren't uncommon.

Mascara is another eye makeup, basically to increase eyelash length and diameter. Most mascaras are a combination of wax or soap with non-permanent color pigment added. Cakes are usually moistened with water before the mascara is brushed on. Creams often come in tubes, but are also applied with a brush. Liquid mascaras generally come with self-applicators. The latter is the most water-resistant. Mascara is generally colored brown or black, but our fellow who opts for a shimmering green highlighter might just flip for kelly green mascara. Get the butterfly net.

Rouges? Lipsticks? Artificial beauty marks? What can I tell you? Foundation makeup makes some sense, since it protects the skin. Yet, today, any opaque makeup is for the man who hears a different drummer. Few are ready to strike up a fully-orchestrated makeup band.

But before this discussion takes a bad turn, here's one pertinent fact: Most male transvestites are heterosexual. Enjoying dabbling with makeup does not a gay man make. And who the hell cares anyway? Only voyeurs are obsessed with anyone else's bedroom habits.

Eye makeup should never be removed and reapplied repeatedly at one setting. Don't use any cosmetics on the borders of the eyelids, inside the lashes; this can lead to eye irritation and blurring of the vision, not to mention the permanent staining of the conjunctiva (the membrane lining the inner surface of the lid and the exposed surface of the eyeball).

Makeup must be carefully and scrupulously removed to avoid contamination by skin waste, bacteria, and environmental debris. If soap and water won't remove the cosmetics, but cold cream will, this fact says something about the amount of makeup applied. Cold cream is a mainstay in the theatrical dressing room.

CHAPTER 16

JOB OPENINGS
FACIAL ORGANS

Anatomically, eyes, ears, nose, and mouth are all differentiated organs to accomplish the work of seeing, hearing, smelling, and eating. Aesthetically, their physical relationship to one another creates the overall impression of a face's attractiveness. When most people think about proper care for the face, pampering the skin usually hops first to mind. But facial organs need some loving, too.

ON A CLEAR DAY
EYES

If eyes are the mirrors of the soul, a lot of souls suffer constant embarrassment. Blurry, red eyes give a depraved look, and their cause is probably deprivation of sleep and/or incontinent consumption of booze, cigarettes, or drugs. Also contributing to the appearance of morning-after eyes are ill-fitting glasses and diseases that include bacterial or viral infections of the eyes themselves and generalized health problems, such as respiratory ailments and rhumatoid arthritis.

Assuming tired, reddish eyes are the result of overindulgence, the condition should remedy itself within a day if the eyes are healthy. Normal eyes are best left to their own devices—in this case, tears, though not necessarily of Wailing Wall intensity—to soothe themselves. Eyewashes have been termed "among the least helpful" of all over-the-counter drugs sold. Yes, they do produce a *brief* soothing, and that's about all. Although drops or baths that claim to get the red out also accomplish the feat, unfortunately a rebound effect follows, so that when the redness returns, it comes back with a vengeance. Repeated usage of these products leads to more frequent and increasing dosages to "clear up" the difficulty. Worse, constant use of eyewashes, drops, and baths may blind someone to chronic eye problems, among them glaucoma, a disease that can cause literal blindness.

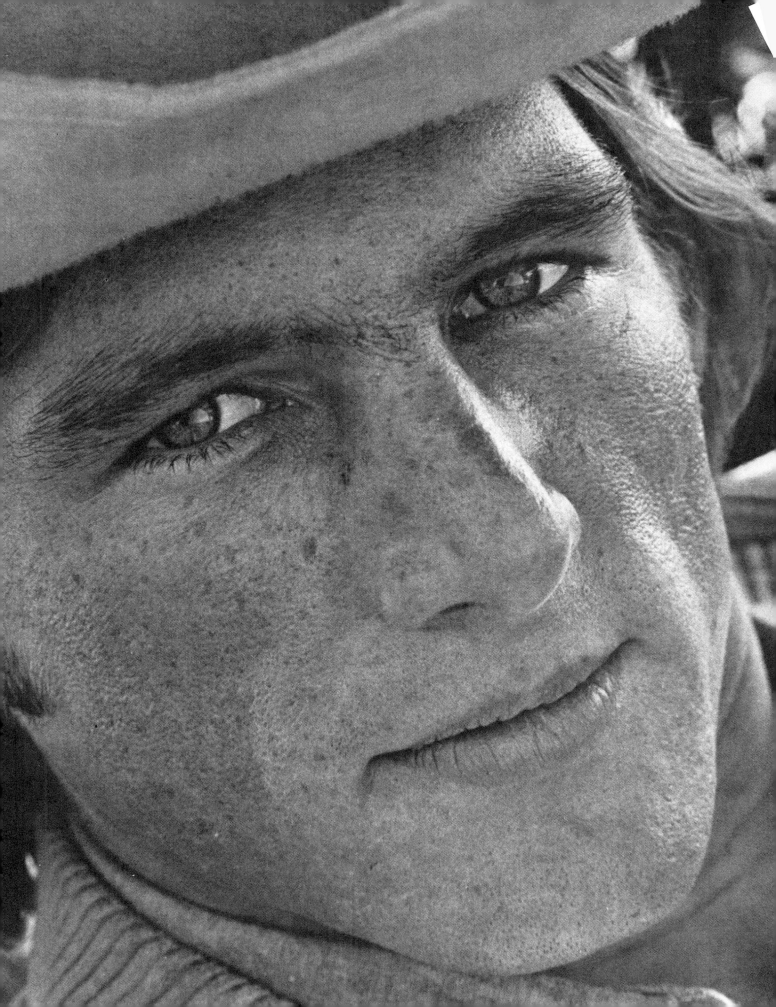

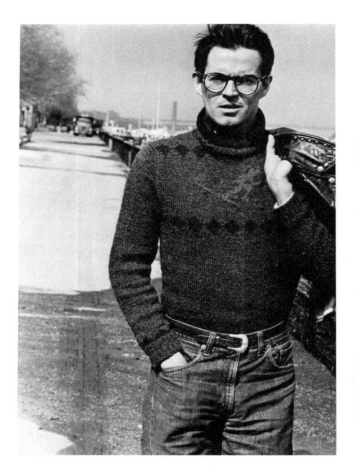

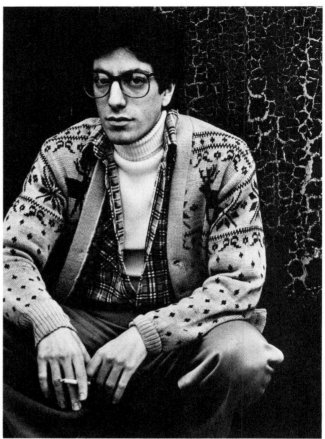

If tired, blurry eyes demand some pampering, first the cause should be removed. On one of *those* days, though, home remedies are safer and cheaper. The simplest is placing one or two drops of cold tap water in the lower lids with a clean eye dropper, closing the eyes, and letting natural tearing wash away the discomfort. Adding a teaspoon of salt to a pint of water (boiled and cooled to room temperature), then dipping cotton pads into the water and placing them on the closed eyelids for about five minutes is also very refreshing. So are cold fifteen-minute compresses on the eyelids.

Never rub eyelids with your fingers. Though remarkably hardy, eyes are nonetheless highly susceptible to infection. If you must rub, gently use a clean tissue. Smarting, burning, itching, and inflamed eyes and eyelids usually indicate an infection or an allergic reaction. Bacterial infections are usually simply cured, if diagnosed, by antibiotic drops or ointments.

Bags and dark circles under the eyes are often hereditary, although lack of rest never helps. Puffiness and darkening likewise advance with age. That's because the skin beneath the eyes is thinner and more delicate than anywhere else on the body. Since this skin is loosely attached to begin with, when underlying muscles and tissues are damaged or lost, the lower lids sag into the openings. Then some of the fatty tissue beneath the skin pushes through the degenerated muscles, puffing the inflated skin back out. *Voilà,* bags.

Dark circles, on the other hand, are, as stated, supposedly no more than the consequence of blood passing through the veins close to the thin surface of the eyelids. These are accented when you're tired or physically weakened. There's little you can do other than cover them with a light smear of skin-toned makeup. Tinted glasses make dark circles less noticeable.

FRAMED
CORRECTIVE LENSES

Repairing faulty vision is mandatory. Living in a constantly blurry haze may at times seem pleasant—

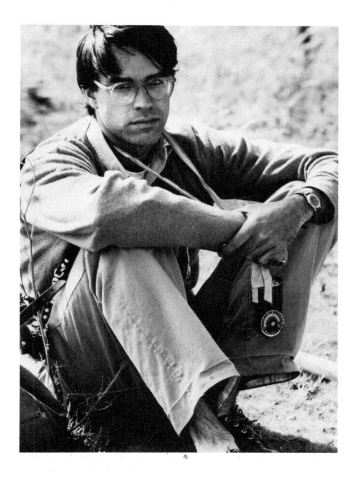

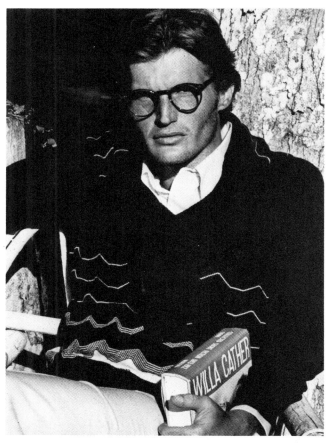

we can transform the world into our private visions—but mainly we're left with our defenses down. Facing reality may be the pits, but what we don't see *can* hurt us.

Obviously, vision is not a grooming consideration. But since some men must wear corrective lenses almost all the time (except during the most private moments), glasses can be as integral to someone's appearance as his hair or skin.

The choice between contact lenses in their various forms and glasses in their varied framed shapes must be personal. Some individuals simply can't adjust to contacts but must wear spectacles. Others experience no discomfort from contacts but have severe headaches after donning even lightweight frames for only a short time.

Ironically, glasses frames have become so fashionable that many contact lenses wearers purchase uncorrective glasses simply for the look. Sunglasses cut down the glare of light while protecting eyes from windblown particles in the air. Lightly tinted glasses can be worn constantly without straining the eyes, but truly dark sunglasses are best worn

only in the sun. Wearing sunglasses indoors makes a man look as if he is hiding behind a psychological screen. The perception of the world around us is off-base when seen perpetually gray.

Choosing glasses frames is necessarily idiosyncratic, since such a plethora exists. To know how you'll look in particular spectacles, you must try them on. A few (admittedly very loose) guidelines exist.

Rimless: Of course, these frames aren't really rimless, or you'd be struggling with two monocles. But the frame is so frail it seems to disappear. This type frame is very stylized, a bit reminiscent of Erich von Stroheim. Since the roundness of the lenses is emphasized, someone with a pudgily round face should never consider them. Strong cheekbones and a cleft in the chin are accented to advantage.

Goggle Look: The antithesis of the rimless frame. Broad and brawny gogglelike glasses can camouflage eyes that are too closely set. They can also overpower thin faces. But if the face is widely flat, this style emphasizes the shape. Having lower bridges, these frames shrink largish noses somewhat. When the frames are very dark, gogglelike glasses are tricky if the hairline is low, better when the hair is receding or combed off the face. But they are a bit extreme. Don't rush into this style.

Square Frames: These also disguise eyes set very close together; and they can likewise look a bit eccentric. Bad for a square chin, the frames offset either pointed or round chins.

Schoolboy Horn-Rims: Perhaps a little unsophisticated. However, if your self-image is conservative-to-staid, these traditional frames will complete the picture. Having more vertical depth, they do slenderize roundish faces.

Oval Frames: Good on good faces. But, then, what isn't? Oval frames don't interfere with the focal balance of the face's structure. In silver and gold, they're quite elegant—possibly too elegant for all occasions. In tortoiseshell, they're still chic but more adaptable.

Half-Frames: They impart a stylized look and an intellectual one too. Half-frames are only suitable for the myopic. Terrific on someone with a good nose, bad on someone with chipmunk cheeks, these frames focus attention on the lower part of the face. Fine if the lips and teeth are good. Unattractive with thin lips and tiny teeth.

Aviator Look: A deserved classic. Coming in many variations, aviator styles can be adapted to almost every facial configuration. When they have greater depth near the nose than at the temples, widely set eyes are downplayed or a Roman nose is played up. The high-setting bridge makes pug noses look less insignificant. Too long noses, however, appear longer.

Elton John Types: If you're a superstar, why not? Otherwise, think thrice.

Generally someone with pallid coloring looks better in metal or lightly colored frames, since heavy black, for example, draws too much attention to the frames. Clear or silver-gray plastic frames look good on a man whose hair is graying, especially prematurely. Silver metal frames are colder than gold. Blue or yellow tinted lenses are distinctive, no doubt, but soft rosy beige covers bags and circles better. To repeat, other than these rather simple rules, trying on a variety of spectacles is the only way to know for sure what suits you.

FRONT & CENTER
THE NOSE

There it is, center stage on your face, for all the world to see. If it's a star, take a bow. If it makes you want to retreat to the wings, try camouflaging it with an appropriate hairstyle (see Chapter 2) or consider plastic surgery. If it's ho-hum, live with it. One must not, however, live with protruding hairs bristling from the nostrils. Hair within the nose has its functions. It slows down incoming air and adjusts its temperature before it can gust inside. Nasal hair also traps airborne debris while inhibiting mucous from dripping over the lips. Hurrah for hair *inside* the nose! But when it presents itself outside, it's ready to be clipped. Don't yank or pluck. The lining of the nose is too sensitive for that. And don't use scissors with sharp points. Moustache scissors are often perfect for trimming unwanted nasal hair.

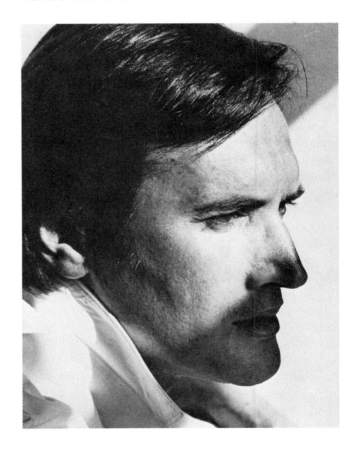

Also unwanted on the nose is excessive oil. Since sebaceous glands are so plentiful there, the nose may often appear greasy while the rest of the face does not. In that case, avoid oily lotions or creams on the nose. If your nose requires degreasing two or three times a day, do it. Many astringents come in handy little packets expressly for this purpose. But if the cheeks are normal, leave them alone. And don't spread the astringent pads onto the delicate skin under the eyes.

Excessive redness of the skin can be caused by broken capillaries, which may be quite pronounced on a prominent nose. Sometimes the central area of the face is dilated by small blood vessels, indicating rosacea, a disease whose cause is unknown. Heightened by emotional unrest, exposure to climatic extremes, and by spicy food and strong drink, it is treated differently depending upon severity. Tranquilizers may help. So may some antibiotics. A nose like a cherry should be examined by a dermatologist.

Another nose dilemma is rhinophyma, sometimes called the drinking-man's disease. It's not understood why nearly no women are affected or why it strikes at all. Nonimbibers may also have bulbously misshapen and reddened nasal tips. But overindulgence in *something* (no doubt, something good) is commonly held to be the cause. Understandable worry about the condition worsens it. Medical assistance is always called for. Sometimes the broken blood vessels can be extracted by an electronic needle. Cosmetic surgery is dictated in advanced cases.

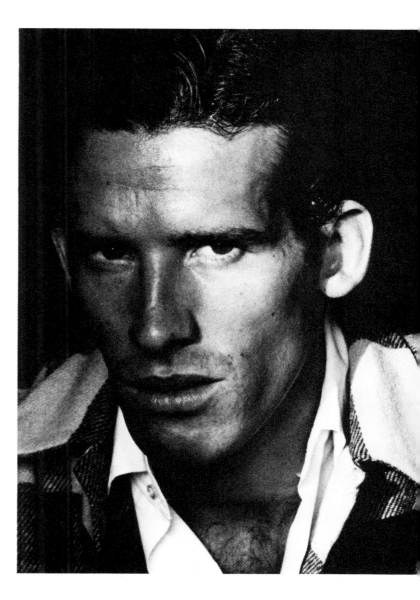

SOUND ADVICE
EARS

Like the nose, there's not much to be done with the ears genetically delivered other than to accept them, to camouflage them, or to undergo cosmetic surgery in order to alter them. Like the nose, when ears become hairy, they should be clipped (the hairs, that is), probably using the same blunt-tipped scissors that you'd use for nasal hairs.

Fortunately, ears are never oily, but they do become waxy. And if the nose is prone to excessive oiliness, probably the ears produce lots of wax, too, since earwax is glandular in origin. It lubricates, protects, and cleanses the external ear canal. At first earwax is soft and oily. But as it gets older, it turns browner and harder. Superfluous wax is removed by daily cleansing supplemented with occasional use of Q-tips. However, if a veritable ball of wax does collect at the inner end of the canal and doesn't budge, don't reach for a bobby pin. Reach for the phone and call a doctor instead. The ear is far too vulnerable to be bayoneted; the eardrum may be ruptured. And don't pour in hot oil either. Boiling miscreants in oil was a medieval torture. Your ears deserve better.

Some men get their kicks from wearing earrings. Self-piercing, although widely done, can prove to be a kick in the head. Although this may seem like a plug for physicians, piercing, either self-performed or by friends, risks complications. Even jewelry establishments and their implements may not be the cleanest. Sterile instruments are crucial. Contaminated ones can spread hepatitis.

Ears are (or, more popularly, one ear is) first pierced with a sterile needle or sharp implement. A starter earring or wire is inserted until the wound heals. Once the opening is thus established, it should remain pierced for life.

LIP SERVICE
THE MOUTH

To most Americans, halitosis is a condition worse than leprosy. If bad breath is persistently longstanding, it can indicate decaying teeth, diseased gums, or extended breathing through the mouth due to nasal blockage. Remember how when you have a cold your mouth tastes foul and your breath reeks. Normally, when the nostrils are unclogged, nasal secretions (which are dried by a cold) prevent the entrance of microorganisms into the system. During mouth breathing, though, these little rascals enter through this orifice and do their nasty work inside the mouth. Even when we're healthy, our internal defenses rest during the night (while bacteria continue to act on our food), hence we have unsweetened breath upon awaking.

When morning-mouth persists all day, many men reach for mouthwashes or mouth sprays to refreshen their breath. Well, these products do help for a very brief time. Not absorbing odor, they mask it. A mint would do just as well. If mouthwashes or sprays are for romance, gargle or spritz and then lunge. As for gargling to remove food particles, plain water works just as well.

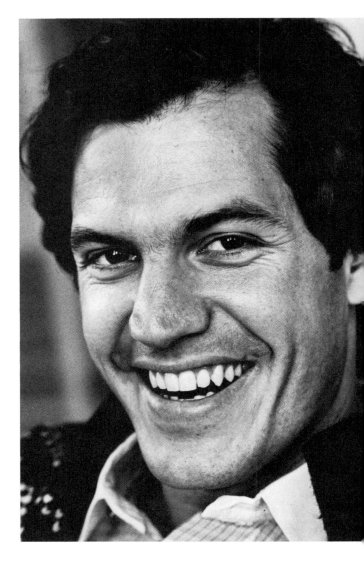

Nor are food particles the villains in halitosis that they're often supposed to be. (They're not good for dental care, but that subject follows.) Garlic breath is seldom caused by garlic remaining inside the mouth. As the garlic-laden food is digested, aroma-carrying materials are absorbed into the blood stream and exhaled through the lungs. Since mouthwashes are relatively inefficient, if you gargle with one after eating, it will have no effect on the garlic odor from respiration that follows digestion. Eating parsley to "eat up" garlic fumes internally before they can be released is a time-honored and reliable antidote.

Chapped lips don't contribute to bad breath, but they certainly detract from the face's appearance. Besides, they hurt.

The best way to avoid chapped lips—or sunburned or windburned lips, for that matter—is to avoid the causes: unfriendly elements that dehydrate them. People with protruding lower lips or who breath through their mouths (a habit they should break) are especially susceptible to lip dehydration. Water-based moisturizers won't protect because saliva washes them away. Oil-based lipsticks suffice for women. Clear lipsticks (glosses) will normally do for men. However, if the lips are constantly exposed to wind, sun, or cold, zinc oxide (that gunky white stuff that looks so ridiculous) offers maximum protection by creating an impenetrable physical barrier. Nervous types should check from time to time to make sure they haven't chewed away their protection.

ORGAN GRINDERS
TEETH

Anyone who has suffered the outrageous fortune of being called Bucky Beaver or Metal Mouth during his tender formative years knows that bad teeth make a biting impression. But even as an adult, our friend can feel virility challenged if his now otherwise straightened and perfect teeth aren't glaringly white, a.k.a. sexy. Poor us, constantly being manipulated by the money mongers.

Teeth are more than simple cosmetic insets. The appearance of the lower half of the face owes much to their proper or improper alignment. Even tooth capping, though often cosmetically motivated, is too specialized and too individual to be discussed generally.

Tooth brushing is another matter. Being bidden to "whiten" our teeth by using this toothpaste or that, we can really only do so much. Whiteness or yellowness is inherited. White teeth can become yellow through neglect, but naturally yellow teeth won't become whitened with even the best of care.

Happily, keeping teeth looking their best also helps keep them and the gums their healthiest. The first step in teeth care is brushing.

Many adults discard the brush-after-every-meal theory of teeth care as childish and adopt a morning and evening routine. The folly of age. Brushing before going to bed is considerate. Brushing upon rising helps rid morning-mouth temporarily. But while the gums are stimulated whenever teeth are brushed, lacking in the morning/night routine are the benefits of fighting tooth decay.

Usually attributed to fermentation of sweets and carbohydrates on the teeth, decaying force begins immediately and becomes most potent from fifteen minutes to half an hour after sugar has coated the cracks and crevices of the teeth. When sugar is unremoved, harmful acidic action eats away at the enamel of the teeth. Not childish at all, brushing after every meal is sensible. When brushing is impracticable, the mouth should at least be rinsed thoroughly with water to flush away as many food particles and as much soluble sugar as possible. Dietary control of sugar intake is another obvious assist.

While fighting decay, brushing also helps remove unsightly calculus and plaque from the teeth, which can discolor the enamel (unattractive) and cause gum diseases (unhealthy). As a practical matter, it's not always easy to brush away substances in the nooks and crannies between teeth. Dental floss reaches where a brush can't; flossing daily is highly recommended. (The use of water-flushing machines also helps remove devious food but should never be used to the exclusion of brushing or flossing.) When plaque is unremoved, small colonies of bacteria breed within it, contributing to decay since these little buggers convert sugar-rich food residues into the acids that attack the mineral content of the teeth.

Some toothpastes are more abrasive than others. Tooth powders are the most abrasive. When gums are sensitive, gentler dentifrices are better. None will affect teeth whiteness, since they don't contain bleaches, but any dentifrice will brighten teeth by heightening their polish. The more abrasive, the more brightening. Warning: Too much continual abrasion can be hazardous to the longevity of your enamel.

Swollen, inflamed, or receding gums are not only unattractive but may signal periodontal diseases like gingivitis and pyorrhea as well. More teeth are lost as the consequence of gum disease than from decay or barroom brawls. Bleeding with only slight pressure is a telltale sign that something is rotten in the state of your mouth. Consult your dentist if you have any persistent gum problems; don't wait until your twice-yearly checkup.

CHAPTER 17

THE KINDEST CUT
COSMETIC SURGERY

All men are not created equal. Surveying a crowd of fellows jostling along a busy street proves that males come in all shapes and sizes and that some of the shapes and sizes look better than others. But when genetics hands someone an especially dirty deal, he can bid a plastic surgeon to reshuffle his given features. Although staggering feats of reconstruction have been performed on mutilated accident victims, most individuals undergo cosmetic surgery purely for aesthetic reasons. The primary motivation is unquestionably vanity.

PERMANENT PRESS
GETTING RID OF WRINKLES

Nobody's hot to sport a wrinkled face. Furrowed lines inevitably make someone appear older. Although the cult of youth and looking young has been pushed to whacky extremes, it's perfectly understandable why men want to preserve the best possible self-presentation as long as they can. There's nothing wrong with healthy egoism as long as it doesn't become insufferable egotism. When the face begins to sag, various plastic surgery techniques can lift the spirits and the appearance. (For nonsurgical ways to fight wrinkles, see Chapter 14, "Border Lines.") But people who expect surgeons to possess a secret fountain of youth will have the bitter pill of reality to swallow.

Chemabrasion

This technique quite literally eats away all the outer layer and part of the inner layer of the skin on the face. Thankfully, this destruction is controlled under medical supervision. A caustic gel is spread over the entire face and neck areas, attacking the skin chemically, after which the gel is removed. A fair amount of pain is involved. Two sessions on two successive days may be required. Afterward the skin looks horrible. It may be covered with blood.

Effective in ridding wrinkling around the eyes and mouth, chemabrasion stimulates new skin growth by removing the older layers first. Thus, to some extent,

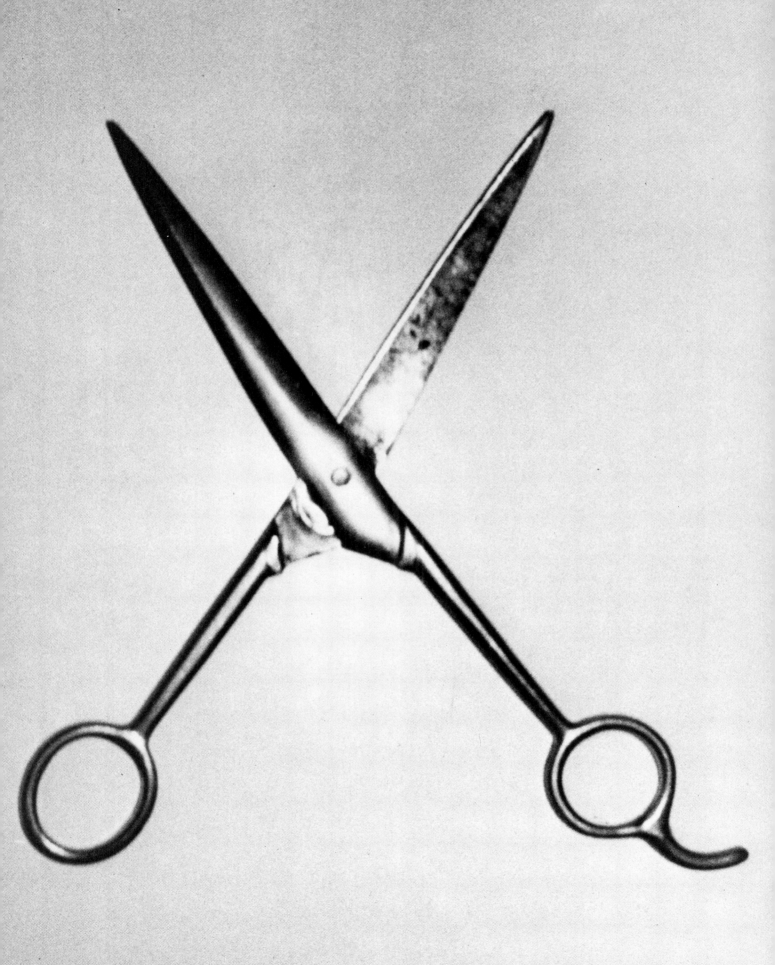

the skin is restructured. Even though the regrowing skin is less wrinkled and smaller pored, much of the new skin is essentially scar tissue. It may not appear as natural as the former, though wrinkled, face.

Sometimes certain areas are more pigmented while others are less so after this chemical peeling. Black skin is especially predisposed to pigmentation discolorations. Since the chemicals involved are so potent, the healing process is slow. Optimum benefits may not be apparent for several months, although a patient can come out of hiding within a couple of weeks.

Dermabrasion

Like chemabrasion, this technique is sometimes used to remove acne scars as well as unsightly wrinkles. It also removes layers of the skin's surface, though with a rapidly rotating brush after the skin is frozen with an aerosol freezing spray. The accompanying pain is traced more to the freezing than to the brushing.

Sometimes called planing, dermabrasion results in a swollen, inflamed face, though the effect usually subsides within a few days. The entire procedure is rather bloody, more so than during chemabrasion, although both result in a scab formation that starts to separate within a week or ten days. Patients normally resume their customary activity within two weeks, although reddish-pinkish discolorations may not disappear for a month. As with chemabrasion, wrinkles and minor blemishes are made less obvious by this upper skin removal, although the results don't always look entirely natural. In neither procedure should miracles be expected.

Silicone Injections

Not only for breast augmentation, silicone can be used in small amounts to soften—not eliminate entirely—some wrinkling. However, after the federal government repeatedly and frustratingly failed to make a judgment about the safety and effectiveness of silicone injections in wrinkle treatment, the only domestic producer of this inert substance in the United States simply halted its production. Since no

definitive decision has been issued as yet, registered physicians can still theoretically fight wrinkles with silicone legally if these doctors have any supply of it remaining.

Some physicians insist that silicone injections, properly administered, are hazard-free. The procedure is simply to inject the silicone under the skin with a syringe. The silicone plumps or fills out the void space that caused the wrinkle in the first place. Horror tales about floating silicone stem from attempts to augment breast size. Injecting too much silicone in soft tissue where it can't be held—for example, under the eyes or at the neck—is courting unacceptable results.

Unauthorized use of silicone is fairly widespread, even given the peculiar shortage. Black market, you know.

The Face Lift

As nearly everyone knows, by making strategic incisions about the hairline and face, stretching the facial skin, anchoring it to facial muscles again, and then sewing up the incisions, a plastic surgeon performs the classic face lift. It replaces sagging and wrinkled faces with smoother, more youthful-looking ones. But not everyone realizes that the aging process resumes the moment the operation is completed, even though the face is puffed and bruised for several weeks. By the time the patient is presentable to the public, one finds that the face has continued to age at its normal rate during the interim.

Certainly face-lift results may be striking, including a certain artificial immobility of the features. No known exercises or creams or whatevers will prolong the effects of a face lift. If the skin is in bad condition, it will degenerate faster. Deeply etched wrinkles won't be thoroughly removed, only tautened by the stretching. If a major cause of the lines has been extravagant use of expression muscles around the eyes and mouth, these will reappear relatively quickly unless the facial contortions are ceased. Some surgeons tell their patients not to smile following face lifts. Humbug. A wrinkled face is preferable to one of granite. Face lifts are fine if kept in perspective. A seventy-year-old man whose face looks as smooth as a baby's behind may himself look like a horse's. . . .

INCISIVE
NOSE JOBS

Thank the gods that finally we're getting over the notion that beautiful or handsome faces must look as if they've been cut from cookie molds. It's becoming recognized that "perfection" can be a drag. The WASP look is no longer the only acceptable one. Still, malformed noses do detract from the appearance. Talk as we will about someone's "beautiful" soul, if we're honest we'll admit that we wouldn't object at all if the beautiful soul were accompanied by a beautiful face. Eccentric noses can be fascinating; they can also be dreadful.

Rhinoplasty

This common form of aesthetic surgery reshapes the nose by changing or rearranging its components. Humps can be removed. Crooks can be straightened. Depressions can be built up. Whatever the desired outcome, the plastic surgeon works like a sculptor. Yet the initial results are far from artistic. Following surgery, the patient is confined to a hospital bed without a pillow; the head is surrounded by the equivalent of sandbags to prevent any jarring movements for a couple of days. Swelling and discoloration are inevitable, but at least the patient doesn't see this, since his or her face is swaddled in dressings. After about a week he or she leaves the hospital, but the bandages may remain on for several days or even another two weeks. However, during this time the dressings will have to be changed periodically, so maybe our friend will catch a glimpse of the new nose—a preview that can be quite shocking. When all the swelling and discoloration are reduced (they may persist for up to a month), hopefully the shock will subside. The artistry of the surgeon—and the patient's own expectations—will determine whether the operation was worth it. It's been reported that up to six months may pass before a nose job assumes its final, permanent shape. Not that it's a floating mass in the meantime. But ice hockey is not a suitable sport when the patient, replete with swollen nose, is back in circulation.

EXCESS BAGGAGE
EYELID OPERATIONS

Ask a group of people what they notice first about someone whom they're meeting for the first time, and odds are at least half will respond, "The eyes." Silly. What anyone notices first and foremost is if the person is female or male. When gender isn't immediately apparent, that's heavy. Still, eyes are certainly way up there as far as attraction and attractiveness go. Tinted contact lenses can change eye color, but only surgery can transform heavily bagged eyes into ones worthy of winning a wink of approval.

Blepharoplasty

Increasingly performed, this surgical technique removes "droop" from the upper eyelids and "drop" from the lower ones. Both excess skin and excess fatty tissue are eliminated. As mentioned earlier, the thin skin surrounding the eyes houses few sebaceous glands, so it is automatically more prone to wrinkles. Connecting tissues become less elastic with age. Fat bulges through the weakened muscles, causing a kind of flabby yet puffy looseness. (If drooping eyelids are caused by drooping eyebrows, then a full face lift may be necessary.) For the upper lids, incisions are made along the normal creases of the eyelids. Superfluous fatty tissue and skin are removed, the incisions sutured. The same procedure is followed on the lower lids, but the incisions are immediately underneath the lashes. After surgery, the eyes are covered with tight dressings that are usually removed the next day. Another day may or may not be spent at the hospital. As in all cosmetic surgery, the surrounding areas look badly bruised. Discoloration and swelling last for a couple of weeks, and the small scars (sutures are usually removed four or five days after the operation) eventually fade; but they are so minute that they're not usually very noticeable anyway. Most fellows feign a sudden eye sensitivity or some other imaginative complaint to explain away wearing dark glasses for a three- to four-week vacation from others' prying eyes. Wraparound eyeglass frames do the best job of concealment.

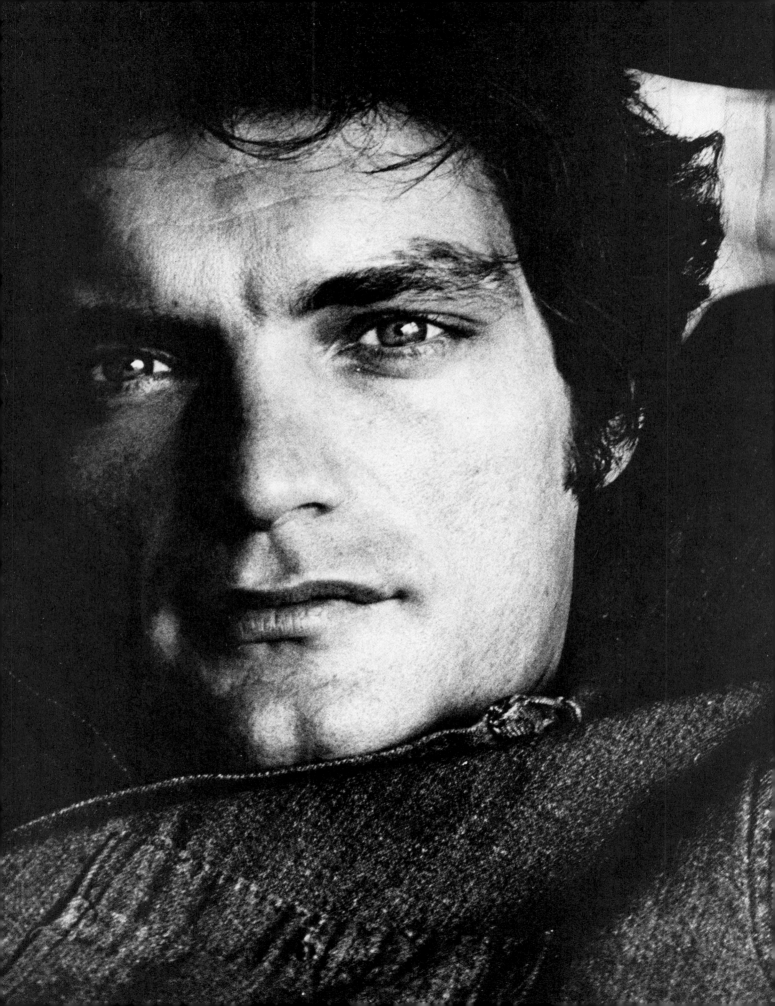

SOUND IDEAS
EAR SURGERY

The story is legendary in Hollywood how Clark Gable flunked his first screen test because some studio yoyos decided that his ears were too big. Okay, they were largish, but that didn't stop millions of hearts from fluttering. Ears may be a marvel of engineering, but they're not the most attractive parts of the human body. On the other hand, gigantic or disfigured ears are no help in looking good. Plastic ear surgery is becoming increasingly common.

Otoplasty

Frequently called pinning and usually associated with children with singularly protruding ears, this type of operation is relatively simple and can be performed on people of any age over five. A long piece of skin is removed from behind the ear and the cartilage is reshaped. How much cartilage is eliminated obviously affects the outcome. The patient is generally released from the hospital on the day after surgery. Pro-gressively smaller bandages may be worn for a week or two, with the sutures being removed on about the tenth day.

Other forms of otoplasty include correction of oversized ears (usually not performed until the ears have been repositioned), during which sections of excess ear cartilage are removed from an upper crevice and skin is sectioned from the lobes.

Ear implants can create otherwise nonexisting ears from scratch. Let's hear it for the surgeons.

SPOT REMOVAL
MOLES

Many forms of minor aesthetic surgery can be performed with an electric needle. Small moles, for example, burn off easily and usually leave no scars, although small scabs will form and last for a few days. Large moles, though, almost always leave their marks. Even viral warts can be dried up and burned away with little or no discomfort.

CHAPTER 18

WEATHER VAIN

SEASONAL CONSIDERATIONS

No season has a monopoly on air pollution, so good skin care is crucial year-round. Keeping an eye on the calendar, if not your face, will remind you that your skin is naturally being influenced by different conditions during different seasons.

THE FRIENDLY SKIES
SPRING & FALL

Don't let the mild weather mislead you. Sure, you feel perkier during these months, but that's no reason to ignore your skin. Nature's gentler course needs a firm helping hand.

One of the most pleasant ways to greet the friendly seasons is by being your own best pal and treating yourself to a professional facial. The relaxation of it will smooth away many a care if not very many wrinkles. Don't get coerced into buying a shopping bag full of the salon's products if you don't feel like it; just indulge your whim for luxury with the facial itself. Do listen to what the facialist has to say about your skin, however. Skin conditions change seasonally as well as over the years, so be prepared to adapt your overall skin care regimen, not only your seasonal modifications.

Of course, you should have protected your face from the detrimental effects of wintry gusts or summery gusto, but if any lines of neglect are evident, erase them. Or at least try to. Skin unshielded from the harsh elements usually evidences fine, superficial wrinkles and lines surounding the eyes, something like nesting crow's feet that haven't gotten off the ground yet. To keep them from becoming true wrinkles, apply a nonsticky oil to lubricate the eyelids and the neighboring skin. Oil is specified because it's more impenetrable than cream, and you need all the help you can get in this delicate area, particularly after it's been abused. Since body secretions protecting the skin are oily in nature, lightweight oils should be compatible and effective. Needless to say, you may not be able to totally rid yourself of these superficial

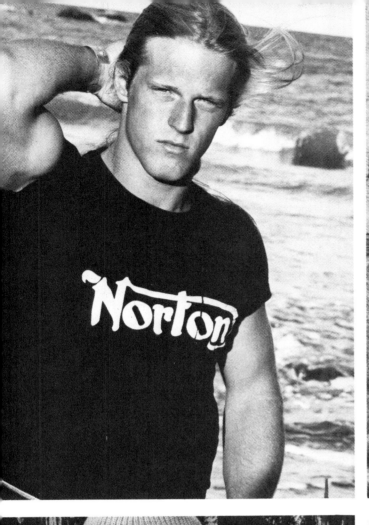
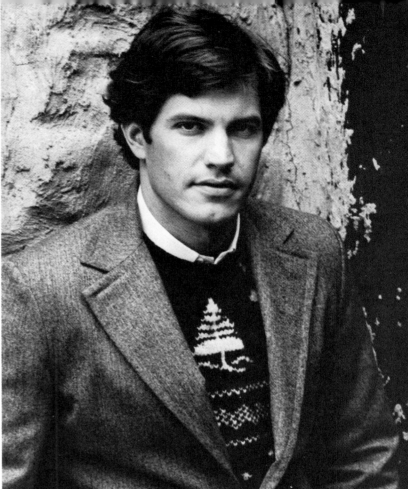
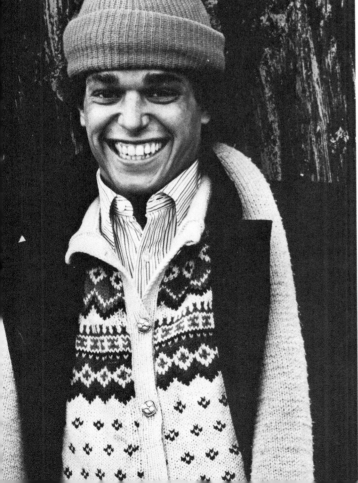
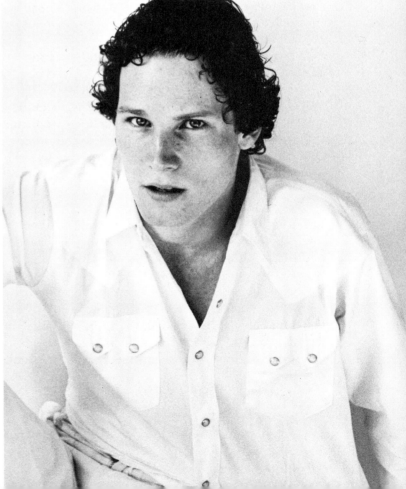

wrinkles, but at least you've tried. After this stronger treatment, you can switch back to a cream or moisturizer if you rebel against oils.

In fall, since facial skin may be both thickened and coarsened from suntanning, you might want to scrub your face with a sponge or loofah (a fibrous vegetable sponge) nightly to hurry the sloughing of the outer cells. Abrasive scrubs two or three times a week, if your skin isn't too dry or sensitive, will counteract the muddy look that often accompanies a fading tan. But avoid the skin around the eyes. And moisturize properly afterward.

Come spring, does your skin look sallow? If so, one professional facialist suggests the following at-home corrective action: Do-it-yourself facial steaming with the herb called thyme. Mix one-fourth cup fresh thyme into a quart of boiling water, stir vigorously for a minute, then, keeping the water at a simmer, lean your face over the steam. (If fresh thyme is unavailable, reduce the herbal proportion by half and use dried thyme.) After ten minutes, turn off the heat but stay over the pan until the steam dissipates. Daily steaming for a week should clarify the pores. Supposedly, claims the facialist, daily steaming for six months helps regenerate new skin tissue. Perhaps. Perhaps not. Admittedly both time- and thyme-consuming, whether or not this steaming really works, a side benefit is that following the aromatic steaming, most blemishes are softened: It's safer to remove them at this time.

Spring is also the time to bring out a tube of bronzer to chase away the winter whites.

Concerning moisturizing: During winter, since you've been (or should have been) using heavier moisturizers and creams to protect your face from the slings and arrows of devastating temperature drops, you will probably want to use a lighter moisturizer protector in spring. Conversely, in summer you've been (or should have been) using lightweight moisturizers more frequently, not glopping more of them on, just using less of them more often. For fall, to simplify matters, you'll likely want to use a slightly heavier moisturizer than you used for summer, while confining its use to morning and night.

One reminder: Don't shove your tubes of suntan lotions into the rear of your medicine chest. In fall, you'll probably still be hiking and enjoying the fresh air. And you can burn during autumn's early months. Once the lotions are stashed away, bring them out early and use them while cavorting in the great outdoors in the spring. Believe it or not, you can get a worse burn in May than in August. Always protect your face. Don't let mild weather lead you by the nose into neglect.

THE COLD WAR
WINTER

Winter's first icy blasts signal rough going for the skin. Frigid air, along with the ill effects of central heating, can cause drying that goes deeper and is more potentially dangerous than summer dryness. In summer, heat activates the body system. In winter, bitter temperatures slow it down, causing the face's capillaries to constrict when assaulted by frigid air. Oil production also slows down. The face can become dry, flaky, and literally raw. Chapping and cold sores may appear as a result of moisture loss. Should the skin become truly dehydrated (when *no* moisture is retained deep within the cell structure), facial skin may never function normally again.

Even naturally oily skin can suffer from the ravages of winter, becoming less supple. But sensitive and/or dry skin faces the greatest difficulties, since neither lubricates itself easily under even the most ideal climatic conditions.

A cheek-to-cheek relationship between man and his moisturizer protector is especially encouraged during winter. However, in bitter extremes, steer clear of water-based moisturizers, which might literally freeze on the face. While you can't necessarily tell whether a product is water-based by its consistency, you can test it by dropping a dab of the moisturizer into some water. If it mixes, the product is water-based; if not, it's oil- or cream-based.

Skin cleansing programs don't necessarily change in winter, but the amount and type of protection applied do. However, fellows with dry skin might want to switch to rinsable cleansing lotions exclusively now. Everyone should still splash his face with loads of water after washing it. If cream- or oil-based moisturizers are used during the freezing weather, remember that they are greasier and stickier. After spreading them on the damp face, wait about ten minutes and double-check. Any shiny or slippery patches should be blotted with a tissue.

Sports enthusiasts, your risks from windburn and sunburn are higher in winter. Skiing is the most hazardous, since sun intensity increases nearly 20 percent for every thousand meters of elevation. Knitted ski masks may look like the devil, but they're heaven sent. Ski goggles protect eyes from glare, and sunglasses are for the sun in any season.

FATHERLY SUN ADVICE
SUMMER

Enough of this dreary talk about how bad Mother Nature is for your face. Happily, some skins benefit from summer sun. Since solar energy encourages the skin to reproduce itself more quickly, it also urges the top layer to shed itself more quickly, thereby unblocking the pores. This increased activity is great for blemished and acned skin. Eczema and psoriasis also tend to improve with sun treatments.

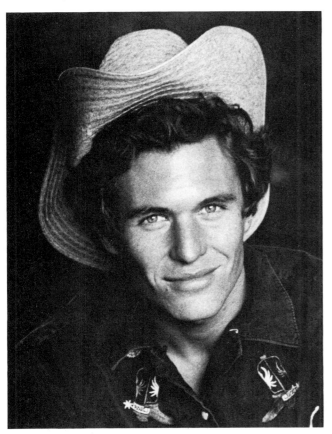

But don't become a Pollyanna about summer sun (or tropical sun during winter) yet. For some medically unknown reason, a sudden exposure to harsh tanning rays may cause an outbreak of pimples, even on people who claim never to have had complexion worries.

Since the sun stimulates the system, more oils are produced. More perspiration, too. When oils and sweat are joined by pollutants in the environment, obviously the skin becomes dirtier than during other seasons. During hot spells, you'll probably cleanse your face more often. Resist the compulsion to overdo; occasionally splash the face with cool water instead. When you do wash your face, be extra sure to moisturize well afterward. Heavy moisturizers are heavies during summer. Use lighter weight water-based ones and even then spread sparingly, forming only a thin, invisible film to entrap the water. After all, increased pumping of sebum affords more protection in summer *if* you don't allow too much sun to take away moisture from within the cells. Guys with dry skin must take extra precautions. No one should expose his face to prolonged sun early in the season without first applying a sunscreen. Don't confine the use of suntan lotion only at the beach. Any time your face is exposed to ultraviolet rays—and that happens when you take a noontime break—burning and drying of the skin are possible. (For a more extended discussion of tanning and necessary precautions, see pages 107–108.)

The sun dries some of the excessive oils from oily skin, but generally not enough. Increased use of astringents helps degrease the face. Don't use them extravagantly, otherwise you can irritate the outer layer of the skin. Wetting cotton balls with water before saturating them with astringents dilutes damaging effects.

As noted, tanning thickens and coarsens the skin. Deep tans are often leathery. Although normally too abrasive for daily use, scrubs can be used by very oily-skinned sun worshipers nightly. (True sun worshipers pay for this idolatry later in life, when deeply etched wrinkles make their appearance prematurely.)

Tennis players who are hooked on headbands court that curious aspect of having an untanned band across their foreheads. They have two choices: either to cultivate bangs or to spread a bronzer over the pale strip.

High intensities of ultraviolet light can hurt the eyes as well as tire them. Sunglasses help.

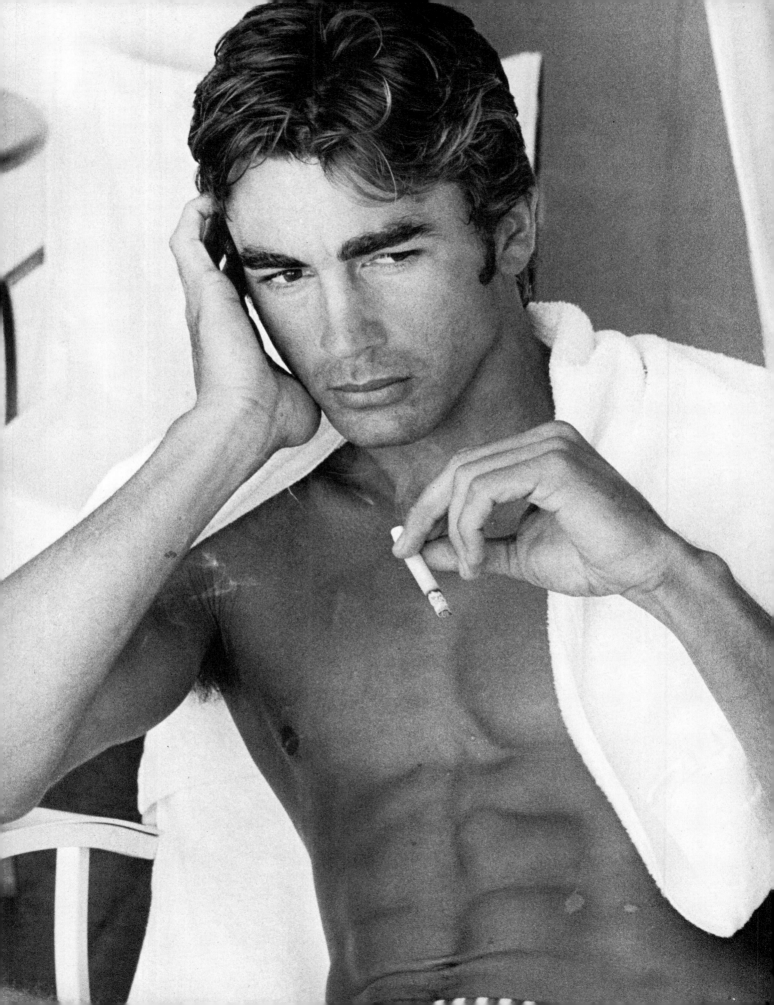

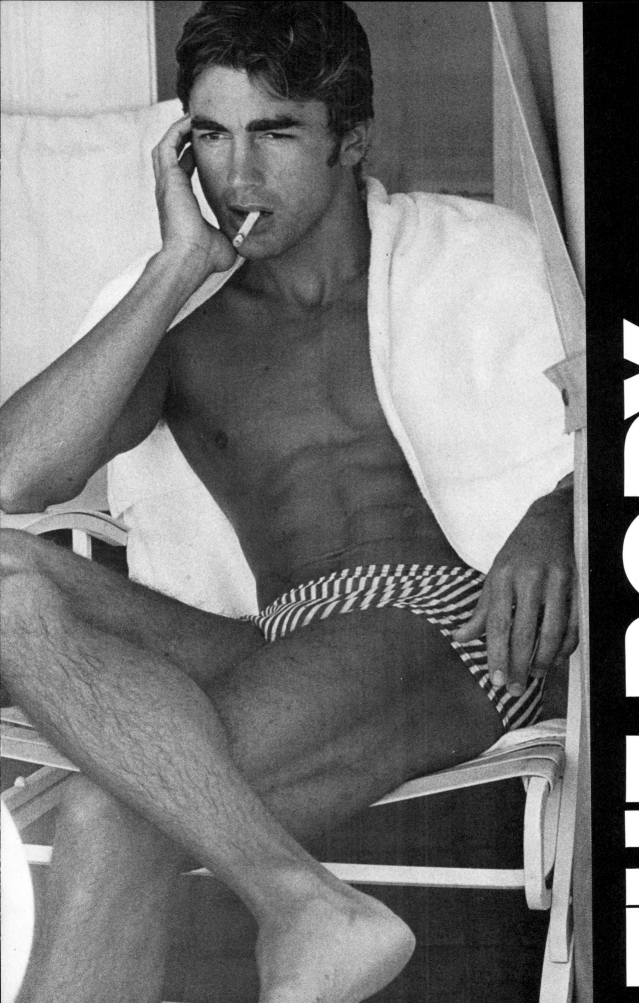

THE BODY

CHAPTER 19

IN HOT WATER

CLEANSING

Look, obviously you need to keep your body clean. But the fear of offending someone can be driven way out of proportion. Why not shift mental gears? Brake any notions that cleansing the body is only our responsibility to others. Relax. Sing a few bars. Buy a rubber duck. Hell, lathering your body is a lot more pleasant than sweating it out in an office.

TUBS OF FUN
BATHING

Baths are supposed to be more drying to the skin than showering. Maybe so. But the pure languor of bathing beats quicker showering any time. Besides, you can take extra precautions—which are kind of kicky in their own right—to ensure both thorough cleansing and protection from dryness.

Bath oils aren't essential to a bath, but if you add them while the water is running, they'll be swirled about and ready to greet your bod. They'll also form a film of protection to fight dehydration (which only oldsters or guys with particularly dry skin need worry about anyway). Foaming bath granules offer less protection but usually smell awfully nice. If you want to scrub with a washcloth, the pile can be richly thick. Sponges, especially those naturally rough, stimulate the skin during bathing and facilitate the sloughing of surface dead cells. Fibrous scrubbers called loofahs make the skin tingle.

O.K. Maybe this bathing scenario is too bubbly. One or two weightier thoughts are appropriate. First, what kind of soap are you using? If body odor is a persistent problem, maybe the soap should be an antibacterial deodorant type, especially for scrubbing the underarms, the feet, and your you-know-whats. However, if you are plagued by dry skin, deodorant soaps may be too harsh. And they're no good for facial cleansing even on oily-skinned men. Although you may resist the inconvenience, it's not a bad idea to have two or three soaps lined up: the strongest for areas where body odor does its dirty work; another

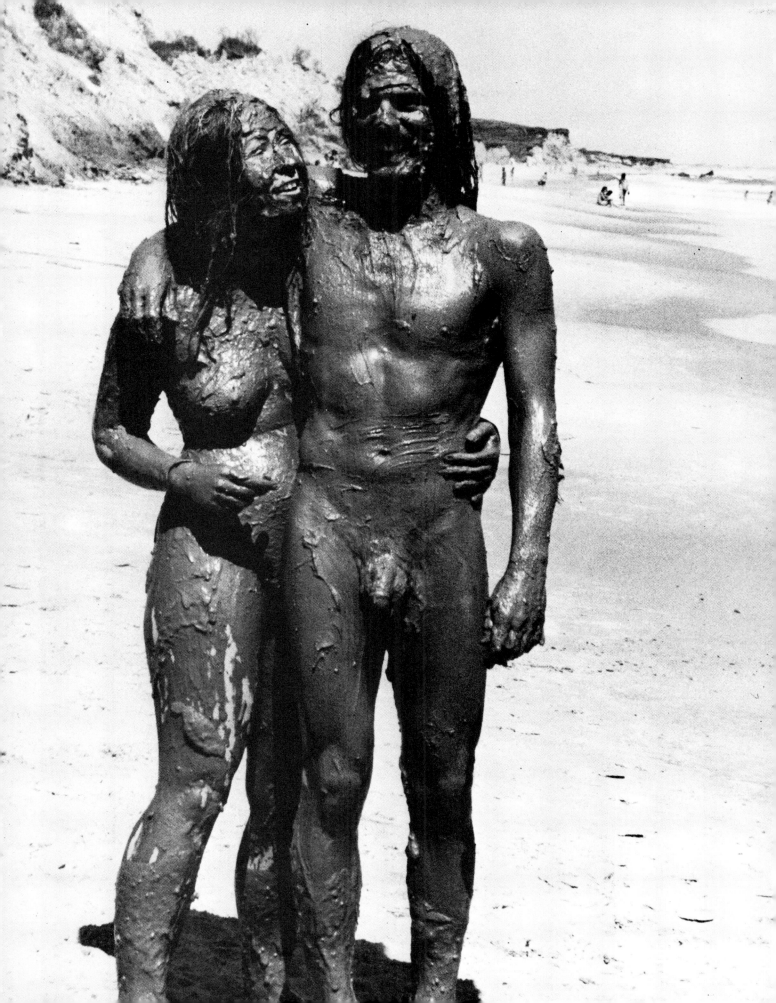

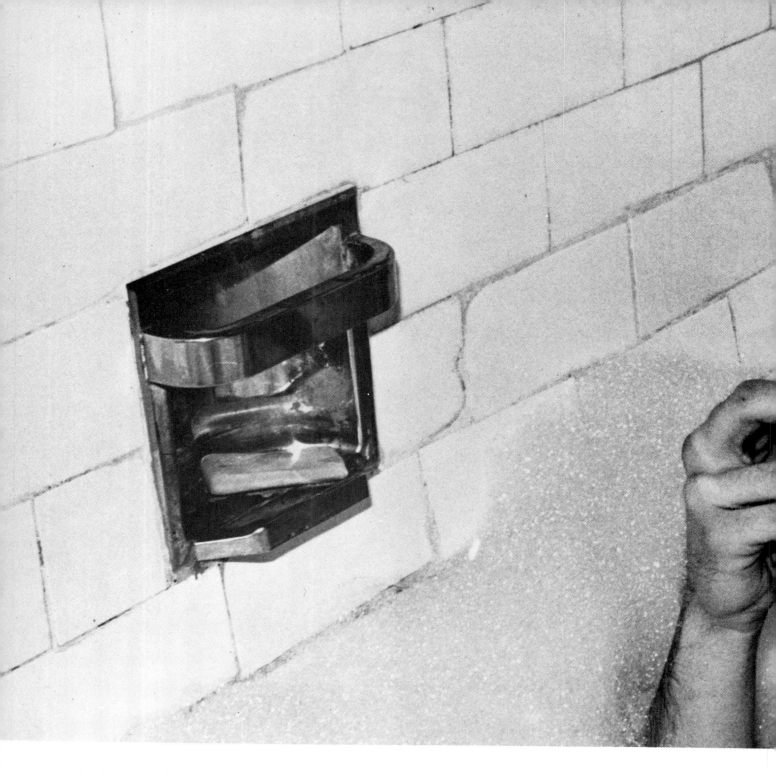

bar (perhaps a fine, hard-milled one) for the rest of the body; and possibly even a third (pure, unscented soap wouldn't be bad) for the face if you must wash your face when you bathe. Otherwise you can save face at the sink.

You probably won't be this conscientious, and your skin will still thrive. But the options are available for the ultimate bath.

Now, back to some more fun. Whistle. Hum. Unstop the plug. But the joy needn't go down the drain. You can make the most of the bathing syndrome by smoothing on a body rub (a scented lotion that lubricates the skin and that is usually a thicker consistency than a body splash—the latter generally being a quickly evaporating, scented liquid to refresh and tingle the body). But lightly towel dry first.

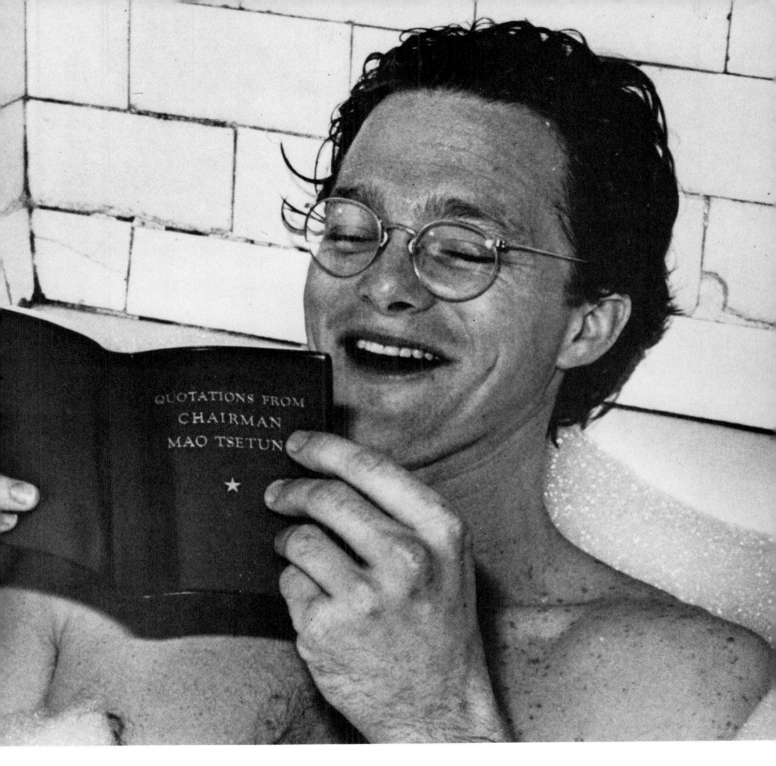

Although you can use any moisturizer, why not indulge yourself? The more enjoyable body rubs are usually opaque emulsions containing emollient oils in an alcohol and water base, plus a fair amount of lusty aroma. The alcohol content causes the product to dry rapidly when rubbed into the skin (massaging is nicer than rubbing, though), producing an allover tingle. The oils lubricate the skin, smoothing it, while depositing a fine layer of protection against moisture loss. And the fragrance may be plain animal. Unfortunately, if you have very dry skin or suffer from eczema, your dermatologist might recommend bath products without alcohol or scent.

Bathing before bedtime relaxes tired muscles, but if the water is too hot, your body may be overly stimulated, and restlessness will follow.

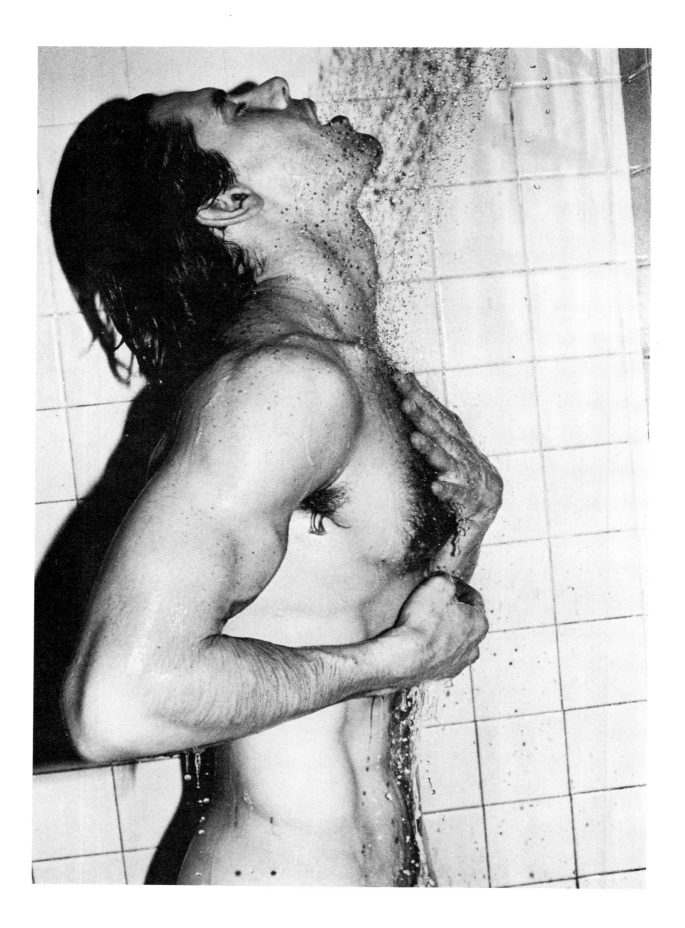

STALLED
SHOWERING

Despite the joys of the bath, showering needn't be a drudge. Two can fit into the stall, too. Lathering bath products are sudsy when rubbed onto bare skins. Sponges squirt. Allover shampoos are also nifty numbers. But the bath question is the same in the stall: How much cleansing is adequate cleansing? Still, don't get tied up in knots wondering whether soap-on-a-rope answers every clean-liver's prayers. Probably whatever you're currently doing is fine, otherwise your nose would have led you to a different body cleansing routine.

Facial cleansing is a far more serious matter than body washing. With any negligence of the latter, the worst that can happen is that you receive a calculated cold shoulder. And that might happen no matter how scrupulously clean you try to be. Caring for the face, however, is ten times harder, since facial skin is constantly exposed. It's unlikely you've ever used a facial cleanser on your buttocks, but five will get you ten that the cheeks on your behind are softer and less wrinkled than the cheeks on your face—living proof that environmental factors are the most destructive to the skin. On the other hand, if you're a nudist, the bet is off.

WHISHING
WATER JETS

Attachments on shower nozzles can whish water in sprays from dribbling to pulsating intensity. Their massaging action helps soothe away knotted muscles since heat does wonders if you're all tied up. Besides being relaxing, these heady implements are great for twosome fun and games. Solo, you'll still find them invigorating. They truthfully won't help you cleanse your body any more efficiently, but who cares?

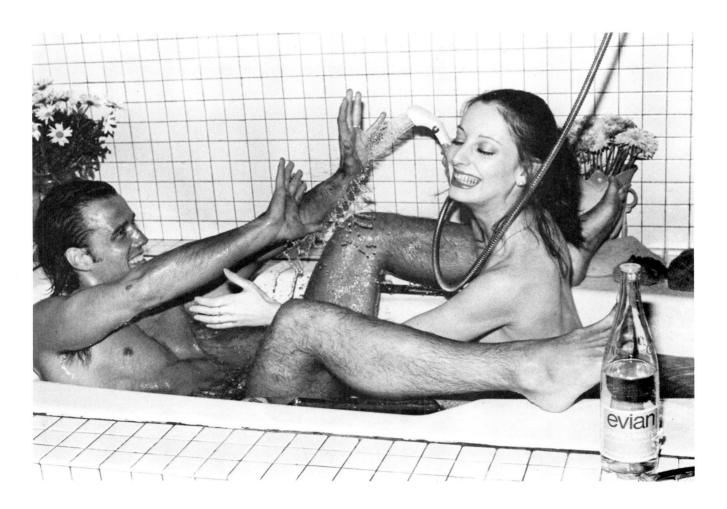

CHAPTER **20**
ON THE DEFENSIVE
PERSPIRATION

If man couldn't regulate his body heat and eliminate internal waste by perspiring, he'd die. So why is perspiration always bad-mouthed? For the nose-knowing reason that it's associated with body odor. Conjectures about the reasons mankind was bestowed with B.O. range from the notion that the aroma of prehistoric man proved so repugnant to carnivorous beasties that they'd stampede miles out of the way to avoid him, to the idea that body odor was originally a reflex mechanism to arouse animal passions among not-too-sophisticated primitive couples. Today, although perspiration is recognized as a vital body function, smelling bad in the process is definitely out of date.

GLAND TIDINGS
BODY ODOR

Surprisingly, perspiration itself is usually odorless. But when perspiration intermixes with bacteria, odor generates. Since odor is most pronounced under the arms and at the pubic areas, understanding the operation of sweat glands in these places versus other parts of the body will make it clearer why body odor is a specialized problem.

The *eccrine glands* and the *apocrine glands* are both sweat glands, but they deliver different types of perspiration.

The more numerous eccrine glands are spread throughout the entire body. Constantly releasing perspiration, these glands are the organism's heat and waste regulators. They also assist in keeping the body moist. Together with sebum, perspiration retards the dead layers of the skin from shedding too rapidly. Ordinarily most men are unaware of constant perspiration. During periods of excessive heat or physical exertion, the sweat becomes apparent, sometimes to the point of dripping off the skin. Since the eccrine glands are more concentrated on the forehead, palms, and soles, these areas are among the first to show the ef-

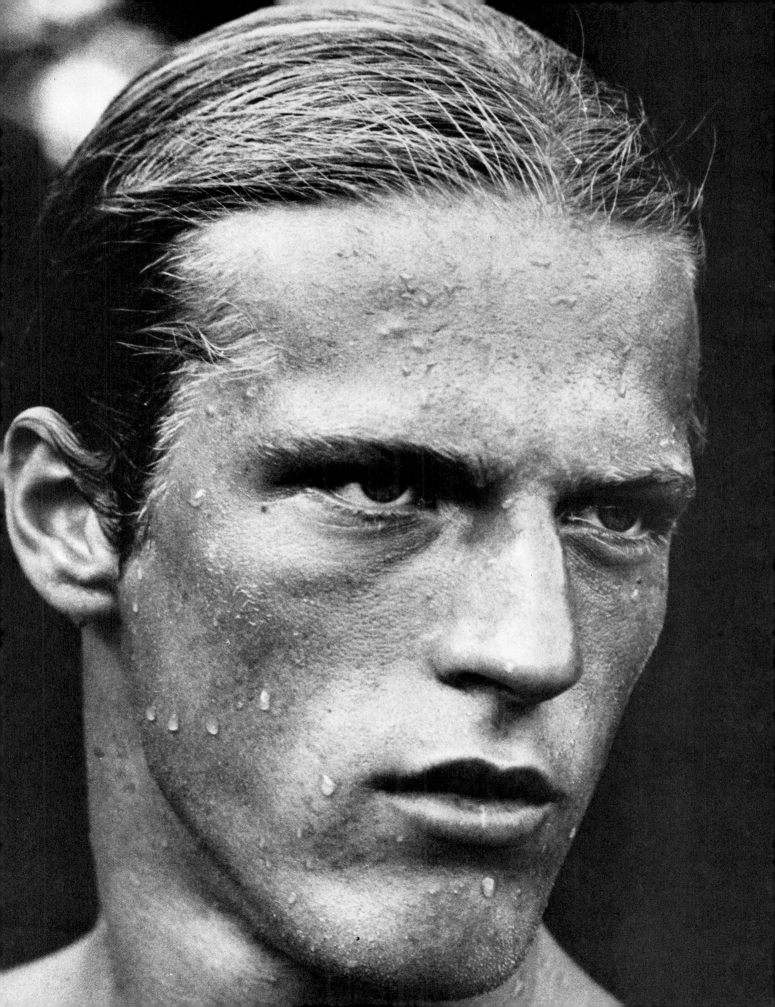

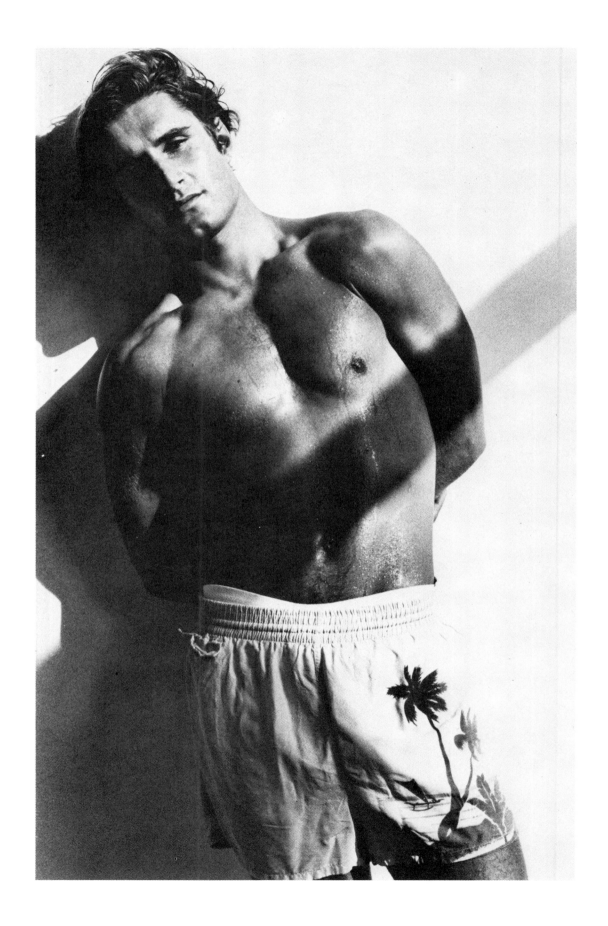

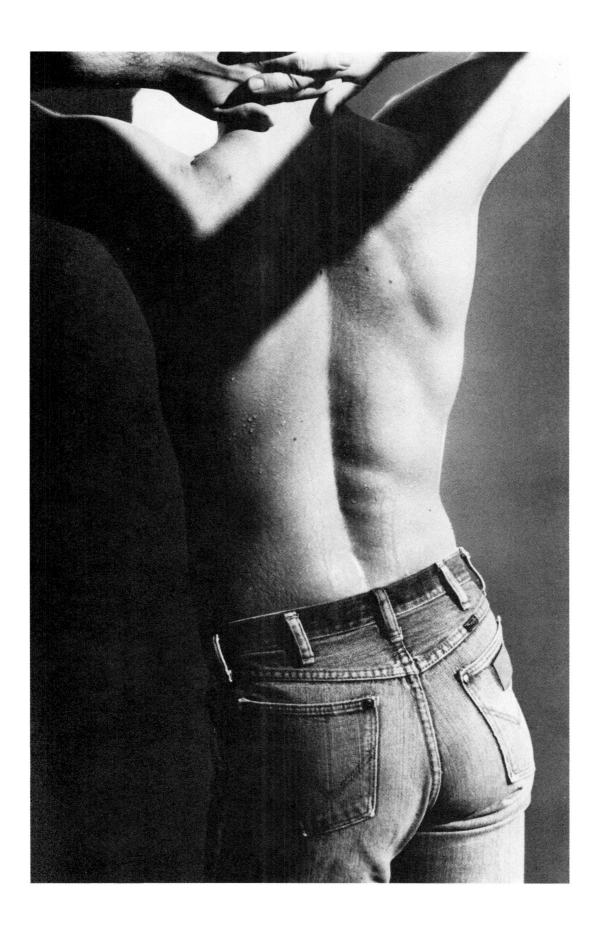

fects of profuse perspiration. Nervous tension also stimulates the production of sweat, basically free-flowing salt water.

The apocrine glands, on the other hand, generally release a sticky, whitish fluid containing various metabolic by-products. Although far outnumbered by eccrine glands, apocrine glands are especially populous in the underarms. They are also found in the genital and anogenital areas as well as the navel and around the breasts.

Bacteria are ever present on the body. But since the little buggers breed best in warm, moist environments, bacteria are at their happiest and most prolific in areas where perspiration can't readily evaporate—the armpits in particular, where apocrine glands are densest.

Although the secretions of the apocrine glands amount to a lesser volume than those of the eccrine glands, when the two are mixed and spread, the milkier substance of apocrine sweat extends its surface, bringing it into contact with more bacteria. The bacteria go to work, and after the passage of time, if the sweat and bacteria aren't cleansed away or masked by a stronger odor, characteristic B.O. is inevitable.

Although the eccrine glands are functional from birth, the apocrine sweat glands, like the sebaceous glands, are stimulated by sex hormones. That's why body odor is seldom a problem prior to puberty and also why it becomes less pronounced with old age.

Apocrine-gland production is more pronounced during physical excitation and under stress. Various physiological and psychological factors affect it. Increased perspiration and body odor often accompany bad health.

Some people naturally perspire more than others. Although, as noted, sweat itself is usually odorless, diet—especially spicy and garlic-rich food eaten in excess—will contribute to odor problems.

Since body odor is the outgrowth of bacteria, and since soap and water can remove these microorganisms for a time, personal cleanliness is the most effective combatant of offensive odor. Since clothing harbors both odor and bacteria, it should be changed daily and laundered frequently. Unclean underwear, besides being an anathema if you're run over by a truck (thank you, mothers of the world, for this universal truth), fosters crotch odor. More about that later.

OVERPOWERING
DEODORANTS

Deodorants are supposed to diminish body odor. Depending upon the chemical ingredients in the formulation, they may or may not. But more often they mask the odor. Technically, deodorants should not interfere with the flow of perspiration. Some do, but for marketing reasons certain companies would rather call their products deodorants than antiperspirants.

Available in many forms, deodorants are presumably more effective the more completely they cover. However, excessive perspiration washes them away. It is questionable that the claims for "long-lasting" deodorants are true if antiperspirant ingredients are lacking.

Deodorants usually have a pronounced fragrance. In order for fragrance to be incorporated into any product, alcohol is inevitably present. So are fixatives. While seldom harmful in aftershaves or colognes, the fragrance imparters, combined with other chemicals in deodorants, can be harsh enough to sting, a sure sign that the skin is being superficially irritated. That is why repeated application of deodorants throughout the day is never recommended. Deodorant rashes are not uncommon. If they occur, the product should be immediately discontinued.

It's hard to justify an argument for hairy armpits, other than supposed masculinity. Since hair holds odor, and most of the odor created in the armpits is hardly pleasurable, B.O. would be more easily controlled if men shaved their underarms. However, the likelihood of fellows doing so is minuscule. And rightly so. Some "irrational" hangups are inescapable if men want to feel manly.

SWEAT STOP
ANTIPERSPIRANTS

Emotions play a large role in perspiration. Worrying about B.O. can contribute to it, so the cycle becomes vicious. Merely applying an antiperspirant can cause the nervous system to start pumping more sweat: Using one suggests how desperately one needs to. Panic.

Some type of aluminum salt to delay the delivery of

perspiration to the skin's surface is common to all antiperspirants. Whatever the products' price, their active ingredients are similar. Fragrance and form are the most evident variables. But that doesn't mean all antiperspirants are the same. The percentage of ingredients will vary. Creams and roll-ons reportedly give more protection than aerosols, although judgments are fairly subjective, since men perspire at different rates and at different times.

Although called antiperspirants, fortunately these products don't stop all sweating. Immediately after application, if they even reduce the flow of perspiration by a half, that's monumental. Most provide far less control. Despite the claims, it's dubious whether any antiperspirants work full force for more than several hours. Their effectiveness decreases as temporarily checked perspiration gets pumped once again, diluting the product in its course. Rebound effects, with perspiration redoubling its efforts once uninhibited, have been reported.

The underarms, like the scalp, can build up a natural immunity to products constantly applied. Alternating two different antiperspirants with different ingredients (these are listed on the labels) can keep the armpits guessing.

Although antiperspirants are no panacea for B.O., with conscientious cleansing they are a decided boost. If fragranced, they mask odor while outperforming deodorants by postponing part of the cause of that odor.

Most men apply deodorants or antiperspirants after bathing or showering. Certainly the bacterial breeding ground should be washed first, but often the heat and moisture in the air from the shower or bath increases perspiration. The products can be diluted the moment they're applied. If possible, allow fifteen or twenty minutes to elapse before applying an antiperspirant.

One alternative to morning dabs with antiperspirants is to use them before the fun begins in the evening. If a man doesn't completely cleanse at this time, he can wash his underarms with soap and lukewarm water, pat them dry, then apply the product. In the morning he might palm on an antiperspirant talc to absorb underarm moisture.

CROTCHETY
GENITAL ODOR

Warm and moist areas evidence a predisposition to body odor. And the scrotum is undeniably a hot spot. But antiperspirants aren't designed for the crotch. The aluminum salts are just too irritating here. Cleanliness is also the key to deodorizing the privates. Talcs help by absorbing moisture, at least for a time, thereby inhibiting bacterial growth. Tight underwear activates perspiration. Probably wearing none is better. But what about mother's runaway truck and your exchange of attire for a hospital gown? Ah, doubly embarrassing. Besides, unlined tweed trousers scratch like hell.

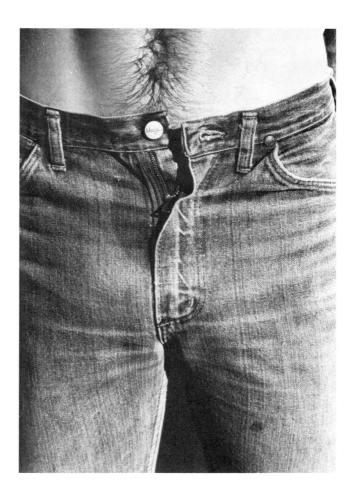

CHAPTER 21

USING GOOD SCENTS

FRAGRANCE

Conditioned to suspect that smelling swell somehow isn't masculine, some fellows underestimate the power of fragrance on themselves by relegating it only to an adjunct of shaving. Foolish. Fragrance, in its many forms, is a pleasurable experience unto itself both for oneself and for others.

LIQUID ASSETS

COLOGNES

A cologne is not a cologne while still in the bottle; it's only a potential fragrance. If you remove the top and sniff, you're not experiencing the true cologne either, since it only becomes "real" or "actual" once it's applied. Then the liquid reacts chemically with the skin. That's why colognes smell different on various men. Selecting a fragrance because it's terrific on someone else makes little sense, since it won't smell exactly the same on you. Oily skin, for example, can change a cologne's characteristics dramatically; and dry skin has difficulty sustaining a fragrance over a period of time. To test a cologne, rub a little on the top of your hand. *Don't* whiff it immediately. Wait for several minutes, allowing the fragrance to settle on and with the skin, then evaluate.

Actually, it's a mistake to confine this discussion only to colognes. In the absence of either industry-wide or federal guidelines to distinguish between fragrance products (aftershaves versus eaux de toilette versus colognes versus supercolognes), all distinctions are a bit hazy.

Despite the feminine connotation of the word, "perfume" is where male scents begin. Perfumes may be comprised of two hundred or more ingredients per scented product. Many of these ingredients are natural oils, also called essential oils, which produce the scent. They are derived from such sources as roots, stems, flowers, grasses, foliages, fruits, and spices. Synthetic aromatic ingredients either duplicate nature's own or add "fantasy" elements not found in nature.

In addition, perfumes contain fixative agents to bind the ingredients, hold the fragrance, and slow down evaporation. Solvents to dissolve the perfume

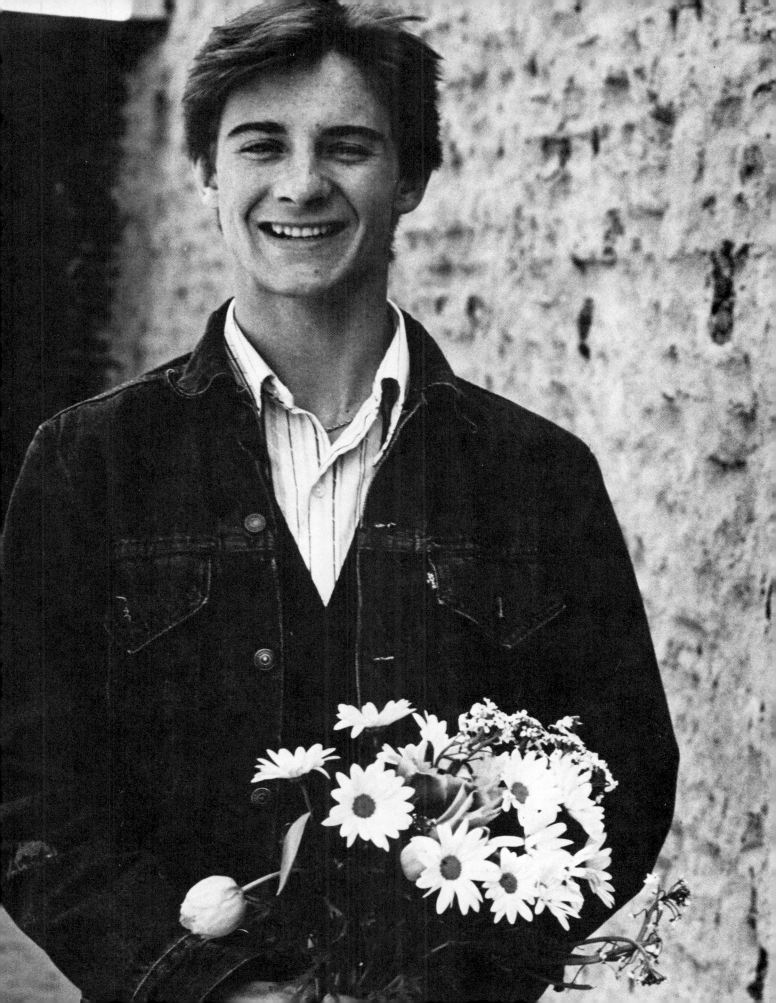

base (the oils) are also required. Since most oils are insoluble in water, the solvent is invariably alcohol; thus, water and alcohol make up most of the perfume's total volume.

Perfume (which is what a so-called men's supercologne really is) is the most highly concentrated realization in alcohol of a particular fragrance. Although no fixed rules exist, the perfume compound might represent 10 percent of the volume. Less concentrated, colognes may only have 2 to 4 percent "fragrance." A standard aftershave lotion is least concentrated, perhaps containing about ½ to 1 percent of the perfume base.

An aftershave lotion almost always has some emollient and healing agents added, but a cologne may not. However, newer products such as "aftershave colognes" contain these extras as well as more essential oils. However, if they are truly colognes, they also contain greater percentages of alcohol and lower percentages of water than do conventional aftershave lotions. The more alcohol, the more sting on a newly shaved face.

These technicalities illustrate that fragrance should be liberated from the shaving syndrome. Aftershave lotions can be *part* of shaving for their antiseptic and therapeutic qualities. Although traditional colognes can work as antiseptics, they usually don't incorporate any healing agents and therefore aren't soothing after the shave. The more soothing aftershave balms have minimal fragrance compared to the supercolognes. Aftershave colognes do have some healing properties, but they don't promote moisturization of the shaved face.

In short, scents-ible men should recognize that fragrance is body adornment, a damned good liquid asset. Fragrance—which seldom lasts for more than several hours on the skin anyway—is more easily diminished if only splashed on the constantly exposed

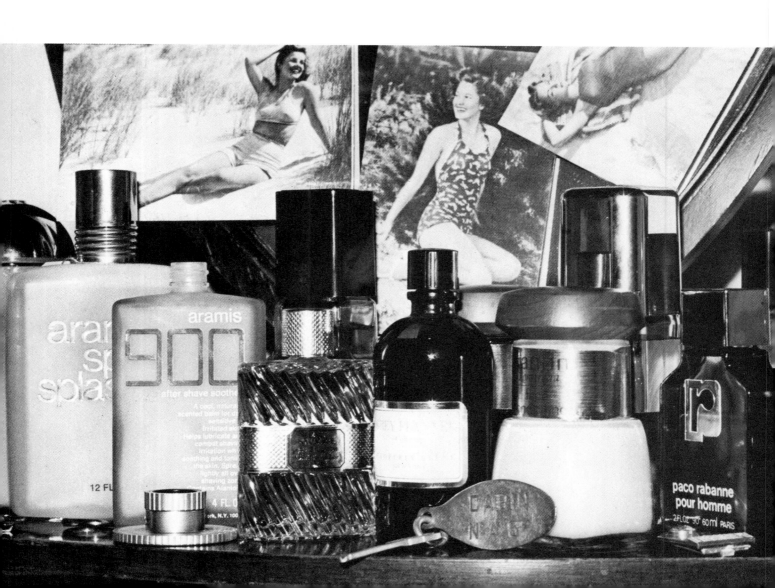

face. Since heat diffuses fragrance, a splash of cologne on the chest, the arms, or wherever you want to spice yourself up spreads the scents-uality around.

The choice of a particular fragrance is entirely personal, since the psychology of smell is very complex. When asked to describe a cologne they like, most men mention something about a "masculine" scent. There's no such animal. What's considered masculine is what's predominantly sold for men. When Billy the Kid doused himself with lilac water, that was manly. Even today Middle Eastern men are strong on heavy, sweet rose bouquets. The fragrance industry is increasingly offering "modern blends"—concoctions without aromatic counterparts in nature. A good fragrance for a man is whatever turns him on, as long as the scent doesn't turn off the individual he's interested in impressing. Unfortunately, no one fragrance has proved to be a universal aphrodisiac. Yet, a relationship between fragrance and sex exists, as both men and women emit distinctive scents of their own when sexually stimulated.

Estimates for the shelf life of cologne vary from eighteen months to four years. But you can never know when you buy a bottle of cologne how long it has rested on the shelf in the store. For optimum fragrance, once a bottle is opened, don't expect it to last more than a year. Deterioration of a cologne results from sunlight, from heat, from oxidation (the air at the top of the bottle), and simply from contamination introduced by foreign airborne particles that can enter the bottle when it's opened. Don't save cologne for special occasions. The harmony of the blend might be gone before you find enough occasions to luxuriate in it.

Light is the most lethal enemy of colognes, so don't leave them near a window. It may not look especially attractive, but consider putting the bottle back in its package after every use. Heat is also destructive. Never store colognes near a radiator.

The most volatile fragrances are the citrus types. These won't last as long as, say, earthy patchoulis. On the skin, it's impossible to estimate how long any fragrance will last. About six hours is considered maximum, even if the dousing is lavish. Obviously, aftershave lotions will linger for a shorter time than a similar fragrance in cologne concentrations simply because cologne is formulated with more fragrance compound to begin with.

Don't mix two or three colognes together to come up with your own private stock. Nor should you splash yourself with conflicting colognes and aftershaves. Fine colognes are well balanced and carefully blended. Mix them and you'll probably concoct a mess. It's been suggested that one cologne can be rubbed on the neck, another on the chest, still another wherever, creating little zones of surprising aromas all over the body. Well, to each his own.

On the other hand, compatible products can be purchased, and these "families" are discussed below.

FAMILY PLANNING
ONE SCENT'S WORTH

Makers of men's fragrance often talk about the "signature" aspect of cologne; that is, wearing one scent exclusively as a form of personal identification. Well, bloodhounds have been pursuing that theory for centuries.

It's far less important to wear the same scent all the time than it is to avoid wearing conflicting fragrances at the same time. Some colognes are sophisticated. Some are sporty. Some are lusty. Choose the scent for the occasion and the mood.

Nothing in this world is truly unscented. Even products promoted as fragrance-free often include additives to mask the odors of the various chemicals. "Fragrance-free" products, then, have neutralized odors rather than distinctive fragrances for fragrance's sake.

In the cosmetics industry, certain companies offer prestige lines. That merely means that their items cost well above the median. Prestige is automatically more expensive than mass, though not necessarily better. Such firms offer products from foot powder to hair sprays, all of which share the same pervasive scent as the line's cologne. The premise is that all these scented products used on the body will be compatible.

There's nothing wrong with the premise. But the strain on a fellow's wallet can be deflationary.

If someone can afford to indulge in a family of grooming products all scented the same, unquestionably doing so is a nicety. If one can't foot the bill,

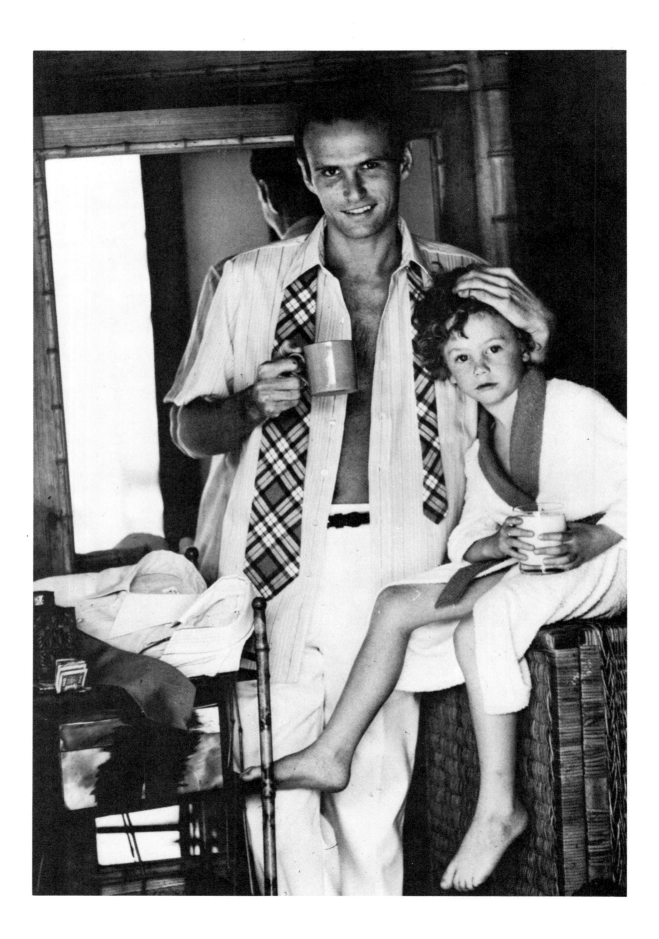

then he should look for neutrally scented secondary products that won't clash with his cologne, which should always receive top billing.

The essential *ménage à trois* in fragrance can be reduced to faithful coupling, depending on one's shaving regimen. For the threesome, the partners are an aftershave lotion (to disinfect the face following dewhiskering), an aftershave moisturizer (to soothe and promote moisturization), and a cologne (as body adornment). The aftershave lotion can be eliminated if a man finds the conventional slap offensive.

Should your favorite cologne not have an accompanying aftershave moisturizer (or balm or conditioner or toner—the terms are mostly interchangeable), then use a neutrally scented moisturizer instead, applying the cologne behind the ears and at the back of the neck, plus on the chest—the same places cologne should be doused anyway. To repeat, colognes are not for faces unless they're aftershave colognes.

If you want to sign a contract with a fragrance, using that brand's antiperspirant (if one exists) comes next on the list. Heat from the underarms diffuses the product's fragrance; the hairs hold that scent to mask some body odor while inhibiting it. If the product is ineffective, go to a nonscented one.

Shaving foam's fragrance is not particularly significant, since any residue should be completely rinsed away. Of course, prestige foams are richer—both in formulation and in price. Talcs, on the other hand, remain on the face or body. They should either correspond to the brand of cologne or be nonscented. For some strange reason, shaving talcs, as soothing and smoothing as they are for the skin, are becoming harder and harder to find. Body talcs can be used on the face without harm, since they also absorb unwanted surface moisture while calming any irritation.

Since hair on the head also holds fragrance, hair products are given the next priority in fragrance family planning. But this need not necessarily include the shampoo (unless it works well and you like it), because all traces of shampoo should be rinsed away. If you use a hair dressing, make sure the scent is compatible or nonexistent.

Obviously bath granules and/or body splashes, if used, should be members of the same family as the cologne. Or the cologne should be skipped in favor of this fragrance alone.

CHAPTER 22

UN-FUN FUR
EXCESS HAIR

Ah, the legendary King Kong. Picture him, the idol of movie buffs as he moons over the virginally shrieking and flailing Fay Wray. Heartrending. While ol' Kong was a marvel on the screen, he just doesn't make it as any man's model looker. The King in tennis whites? Preposterous. For many women, a nicely hairy chest makes a guy look sexy; a hirsute back transforms him into an animal. Sorry, Kong, but too much hair on the body just ain't appealing. Alleviating the problem must be accomplished externally, since excessive hair is usually genetically determined. Shaving is the obvious solution for the face, but nowhere else. Most afflicted men want to rid themselves of some, not all, body hair. Kong isn't their ideal, but neither is a plucked chicken.

PATCH WORK
TEMPORARY HAIR REMOVAL

Scissors: Thick hair, so prized atop the head, is bothersome in abundance anywhere on the body. Dark hair appears even denser than it may in fact be. One of the simplest remedies is to trim and thin the hirsute area with scissors. The clipping shouldn't be performed at skin level, though, or the unappealing shag becomes unappealing stubble. As an example, here's how to trim overly hairy chests. Fluff up the hair with your fingers, then lightly snip the ends of the growth. Absolute precision is unnecessary, but try for a fairly even job: Thick and thin patches draw more attention to the condition. If the chest still looks too hairy, fluff and trim again. Use blunt-ended scissors in case you poke yourself accidentally. A good place to do the job is in the bathtub. But keep the hair dry so you can better judge the results. Then rinse the tub and pour in some Drano.

Plucking: Using tweezers to thin hairy areas is

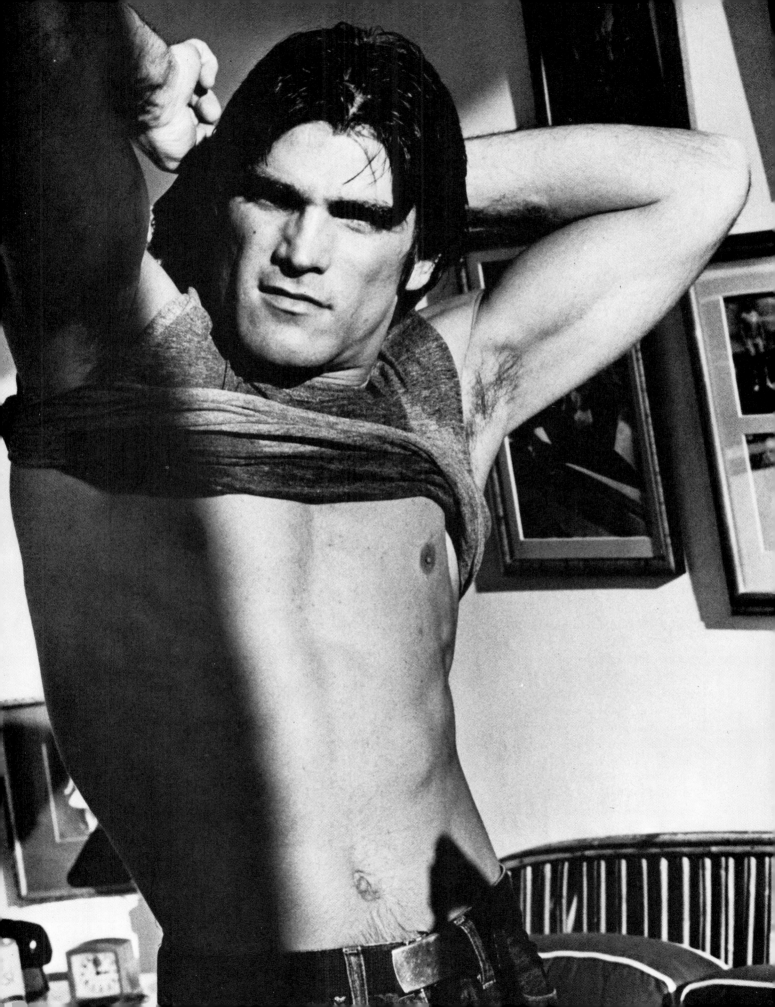

tedious, since you should pluck only one hair at a time. Oscar Homolka eyebrows can be separated by tweezing, but extracting several hairs together is still discouraged; it hurts. Apply an antiseptic after plucking.

Abrasives: Pumice stone (solidified volcanic powder) can rub hair away. Friction does the job. The method is quite primitive, though not bad for ridding too much hairy growth on fingers. Since abrasives act like sand paper to plane away the hair, take care and always spread on a moisturizing cream after abrading the skin. The disadvantages of pumicing larger areas include the large amount of time consumed and the fact that most of the hair is removed at skin level.

Bleaching: Many women bleach facial and body hair to make it less apparent. This technique has only limited application for men. Conceivably, some fellow might bleach excess hair on the shoulders and follow the bleaching with a close scissor trim. In its favor, bleaching is painless and harmless to most people; prolonged bleaching will cause the hairs to degenerate and break. Hair coloring preparations are too costly and too sophisticated for this mundane job. At-home brews of hydrogen peroxide and ammonia (twenty drops of ammonia per one ounce of peroxide) should work but might be irritating to the skin. Commercial facial and body hair bleaches are sold inexpensively.

Depilatories: These products are also more applicable to women, since they convert human hair into a soft, pliable mass within several minutes. Then the destroyed hair is either wiped or rinsed away. Ideally, depilatories should be nonirritating; practically speaking, many aren't. Thin hairs are knocked off faster than coarse ones. Using depilatories on the back isn't easy. Maybe a friend will help.

Waxing: Here's another hair-razing technique used by women, in this instance primarily to rid hair from their legs. Heated beeswax (or some similar composition) is applied in a warmish state to the hairy area. Hair becomes enmeshed in the hardened mass when the wax dries. (In salons, strips of muslin are usually applied to the hot wax, which adheres to the cloth as it dries.) When the wax is quickly stripped away, the captured hairs come along for the ride. If waxing is performed regularly, the hair roots may become traumatized and eventually might atrophy, producing progressively weaker and thinner hair. Waxing can be done on any part of the body, including the shaping of the eyebrows. Remember, waxing removes all the hair entrapped. Depending upon how hairy the area is, removal can smart from little to much. Because the hair is pulled from beneath the skin's surface, the results from waxing are longer lasting than they are from other temporary methods. Some skins may be irritated; all will be if the wax is too hot. Self-waxing on the back might be performed by a contortionist. At-home kits are available; many skin care salons offer the service.

FOREVER FREE
PERMANENT REMOVAL

Electrolysis: Technically, this procedure of removing unwanted hair electronically involves the destruction of the hair papilla (what we commonly call the root) by causing it to shrivel until it can no longer produce a new hair shaft. Practically, electrolysis is selectively ridding body hair from any area other than the eyelids or inside the nose and ears. Types of electrolysis are differentiated by the machines employed rather than by the results.

According to strict definition, the one true electrolysis involves a galvanic (direct current) apparatus. In this method, several needles, in multiples of two up to many, are inserted into the pores (hair follicles) and remain there for a minute or more until all hydrogen has chemically been removed from the cell, thus destroying (hopefully) the papilla.

A variation called the short-wave method is performed far more widely today than the galvanic technique. This modified high-frequency process is properly referred to as electrocoagulation. Only one needle (also called a probe) is used to zap the papillae. Finer than human hair, the probe is inserted into the follicle at an angle that is the same as that of hair growth until it touches (hopefully) the papilla. An electrical current travels down the needle, cauterizing and coagulating the root, thus beginning the *gradual* destruction of the hair cell. (More about the "gradual" in a moment.) Simultaneously, the hair shaft is loosened, so it slides out easily with tweezers.

The procedure is gradual because the root may not be totally debilitated during the first treatment. It may regenerate a weaker hair, which can subsequently be removed in the same method. The length of time to make electrolysis truly permanent varies with each individual, the type of hair, the location, and the depth of the papillae. When hair follicles are distorted (either genetically or accidentally, which reportedly can result from plucking, using depilatories, and various other factors), the electrologist may have difficulty locating the papilla. Likewise, the probability exists that some of the hair roots may lie in a dormant stage, having already shed their shafts before the removal session. Obviously they can't be coagulated and will grow full-strength hair again according to their programming.

Electrolysis isn't completely painless. A stinging sensation accompanies the cauterizing. Some clients take a mild pain-killer before the treatment, but two aspirins should suffice. The hair must be at least a quarter inch long before electrolysis can be undertaken.

The treated area may become red for an hour or two. Swelling seldom occurs, but if it does, ice compresses should reduce it. Scabbing is not especially common. Should barely noticeable scabs appear, however, they'll be smaller than freckles and will disappear within three or four days. If picked before falling off, they may scar.

No soap, cream, facial cleansers, or oils that might clog the pores should be used for twenty-four hours after an electrolysis session. As logic and common sense dictate, treated areas should only be touched by clean hands and even then not excessively.

In cases of extreme hirsutism, electrolysis can be tedious, since it's generally performed in half-hour sessions. To thin down an extremely hairy body, perhaps up to four years of once or twice weekly visits may be entailed. (To repeat: This is extreme indeed.) Aesthetically, when major amounts of hair are to be removed, an overall progressive thinning looks better than doing one patch at a time. The electrologist's artistry is as important as his technical ability. The results are only as good and as safe as the practitioner's competence.

Excessive electrical current can damage the skin. To stay on the safe side, many electrologists are wary of employing too strong a current. While it's a wise precaution, this can mean that the papillae aren't completely destroyed, with regrowing but weakened hair the consequence.

Depilatron: This electrical method of removing hair was introduced in the United States in 1975 in the form of a machine bearing the same name. Hair is removed according to the same principles of standard electrolysis (or short-wave) machines except that no needles are used and the skin is not penetrated. Radio-frequency energy is passed through the hair by a specially designed tweezer. This energy coagulates the papilla, then the hair slides out of the follicle.

The promoters of the machine claim special advantages, among them that (1) the process is less painful since the skin is not probed; (2) it leaves no scars, which can be permanent if too much current is used in other methods; (3) it works on everyone, even on curly- and kinky-haired men, whose hair often sprouts from curved or distorted follicles that may prove difficult to probe with a straight needle; (4) the process can be performed on black skin without leaving tiny white scars, which may result from needle penetration; (5) there are no scabs or worries about infections; and (6) their technicians can work for hours on all areas painlessly, whereas extended sessions with a needle probing hairs that are very close together might risk permanent damage to the skin tissues and could cause localized swelling.

The depilatron method has not eliminated the problem of regrowing hairs. Some critics maintain that because hair shafts are not good conductors of electrical current, more papillae survive than with the short-wave technique.

Whichever electrical method of hair removal is employed, the expertise of the technician is of utmost importance.

When should a man consider electrolysis? If superfluous hair freaks him out, wherever it may be.

CHAPTER 23
FED UP
DIET AND NUTRITION

Strictly speaking, although few people find overweight men attractive, maintaining a fit and slender body is more of a medical concern than a grooming one. Paunchy men may possess well-cared-for skin and hair, but they risk the dangers of damaging disease directly associated with excess weight. And while it's true that good nutrition evidences the happy side effect of improved overall appearance, nutritious eating is a healthy goal unto itself and not merely one for the sake of appearances.

WAISTING AWAY
DIETING

The public apparently has a voracious appetite for fad diets. New ones proliferate year after year, but most enjoy a brief period of popularity only to be replaced by another "revolutionary" or occasionally wacky theory that proves equally short-lived. Fickle people don't want to face the undeniable fact that dieting is no fun. Once the gimmickry and novelty of faddist diets are shed away, one basic truth remains: More input than output inflates. Crudely stated, a fellow blows up like a balloon when he inflates his system with too much unused food.

Although counting calories seems old hat, calories still count. Nutritionally, calories represent the energy released by the body in the process of "burning" food. Food is any substance that is absorbed into and utilized by the body to produce energy and sustain the functioning organism. Some foods (such as carbohydrates) supply more calories and therefore more potential energy or fuel for the body. However, they may have little nutritional value, depending upon their form. The need for calories relates to how active a man is; the more active he is, the greater is the caloric input required to fuel the output. When output exceeds input, weight loss follows, since the body then uses its own reserves of fat to compensate for the calories lacking in the ingested food. Conversely,

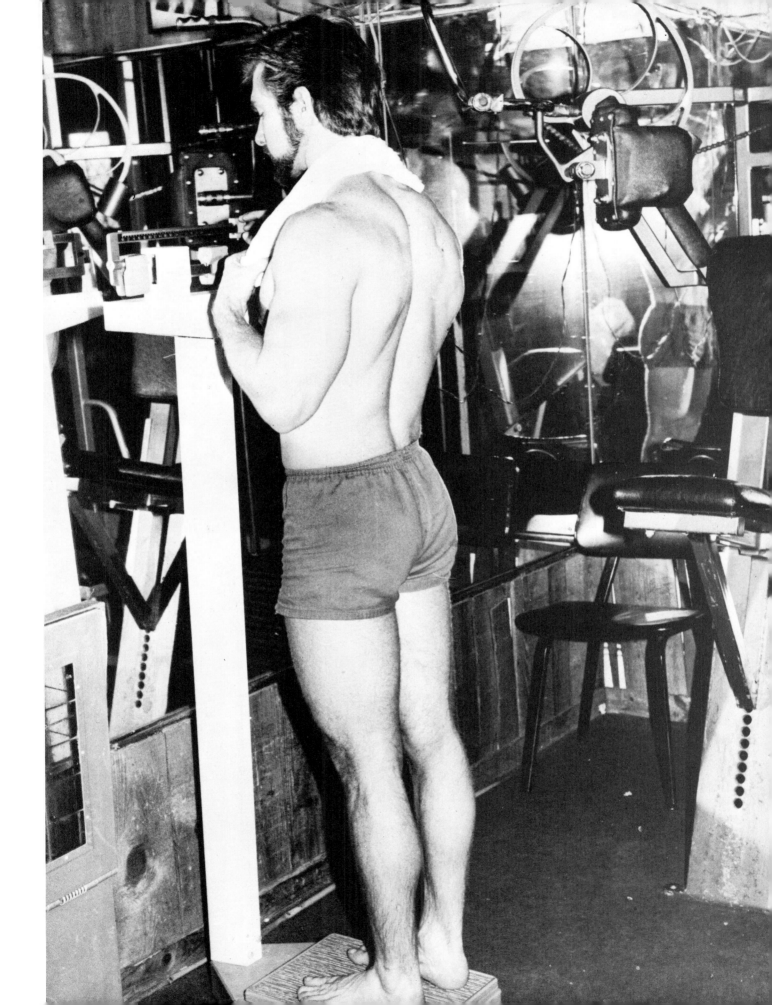

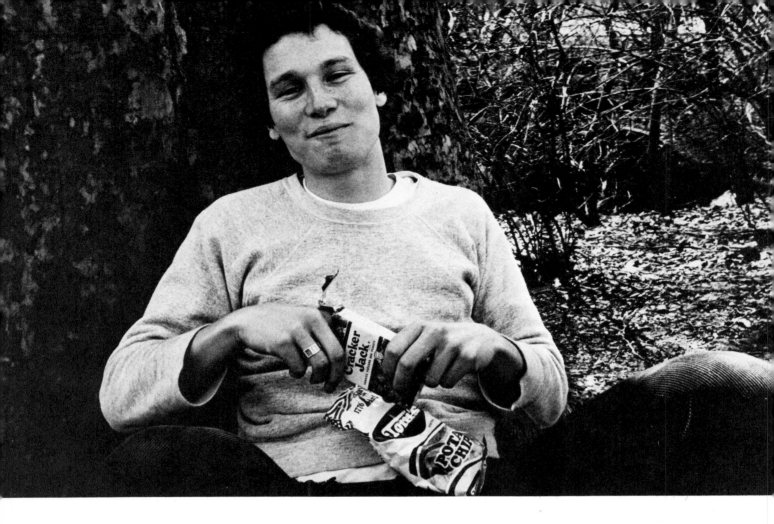

when input is greater than output, the food (potentially an energy source) is not totally utilized and hence remains in the body, building fat.

Ironically, hunger and appetite have little correlation with a body's need for energy and the amount of food necessary to produce that energy. More than anything else, satiation and satisfaction are the creatures of habit.

What most people call hunger is actually the stomach's primitive contractions—reflexes that once reminded our cave-dwelling forebears that they needed to eat to survive. Today, though, self-preserving hunger has given way to appetite, since few people in this affluent society are unfortunate and neglected enough to die of starvation. Appetite is a conditioned response generated by physiological and, more significantly, psychological drives. Unlike hunger, appetite is learned, based on recalling a good-tasting or good-smelling food in conjunction with that soothing feeling of being full. Any food will reduce hunger. But for some, only gooey goodies will curb the appetite. These foods, high in calories, add pounds when not burned off.

Losing weight, therefore, must involve cutting down the amount of calories and/or using up more energy through increased activity. Without additional physical exertion, it all reduces down to curbing the appetite for the wrong foods or for too much of the right ones. It takes a helluva lot of push-ups to work off the calories of one hot fudge sundae.

Many fad diets yield excellent results initially by promising—and delivering—immediate weight loss. But so will almost any form of diet if faithfully followed to the letter, since what's first eliminated is usually excess water. But long-ranging weight loss, and the maintenance of a desired weight, will probably necessitate permanently changing eating patterns. The worst drawback of many fad diets is that they are so horrendously boring that many men won't follow them . . . which is just as well, for some don't supply proper nourishment and can be potentially hazardous to health.

Preoccupation with losing weight—up and down, on and off—can throw the body into a seesaw battle against good nutrition. Anyone can speed up weight loss by eating severely less of every food he enjoys and simultaneously drastically increasing the amount of exercise to the point of risking cardiac arrest. Effective? Yes. Healthy? Not a bit. It may not be true, though it has for years been generally thought to be true, that we require three square meals a day. But we do need a balanced diet.

What is a balanced diet? The difficult answer comes in three easy words: Enough is enough. And enough is when the eaten food furnishes the necessary nutrients, vitamins, and energy to sustain the body and its activities. No more. No less. The body does not "store" protein, for example. What isn't utilized is lost, so eating too much protein is useless. Overconsumption of some vitamins and minerals can activate deficiencies in other vitamins and minerals by upsetting their absorption or storage.

Proper nutrition is far too complex and complicated to be covered in a book geared principally toward procedures a man can follow to look better. However, a healthy diet should never be underestimated. Like so many other mysteries, what is healthy for one man may be unexplicably unhealthy for another. A diet that works for scores may not work for hundreds. Generally, however, if a man is presently in good health and at a proper weight, he should continue eating in a manner that maintains his poundage without fluctuation. If he starts gaining, he should try minimizing slightly the the portions of *all* the food he eats or else increase his amount of exercise somewhat. What counts is the equilibrium, and he should try to sustain this, year in, year out, never subjecting himself to extremes that can throw off the balance of the organism.

Some people who pale at the thought of doing without food or drink (other than mineral water) may find the idea of a quasi-fast—no food at all, but allowances of fruit juices and water—more palatable. But some fruit juices are high in caloric count. Weight loss may not be as speedy as when following the purist way.

RIB CAGED
UNDERWEIGHT

Our society has weird notions about weight. Let someone gain five or six pounds and he or she gets razzed to death. But let someone walk around like a motorized skeleton, and nothing's said. Come on, being underweight is every bit as unattractive as being overweight. Everyone seems to quake at the thought of sleeping with a blimp, but isn't getting it off with skin and bones incipient necrophilia?

Being severely underweight usually indicates a metabolic disorder. Or it can be the result of hell-or-high-water dieting. If it's the latter, the obvious remedy is to eat more and to stop being a fool. That doesn't mean that you should jog off to the candy store for a pound of chocolates. First, the jog will burn up the too-little food you've consumed. Second, chocolate will add calories but not nourishment. Treat yourself to a steak, home fries, and a tossed salad instead.

Someone who eats like a pig but looks like the runt of the litter does himself a favor by visiting a qualified nutritionist in order to find a way to add some meat to his bones.

POPPING IN
VITAMINS POWER

Weird notions abound about vitamins. Some men think that a diet of vitamin supplements can feed their bodies. A dangerous misconception. Without food, vitamins are essentially valueless, since their function is to work in conjunction with nutrients (proteins, fats, carbohydrates, and minerals) to keep the action going. Vitamins are catalysts; they help speed up chemical reactions in the body to create energy and new tissues. Most vitamins cannot be manufactured by the body and must come from outside sources. Food is one source. Vitamin supplements are others. But no food, no action.

Personal needs for vitamins vary. A well-balanced diet *should* provide all the vitamins a healthy body needs. But who consistently eats healthily these days? Besides, smoking, drinking, and stress—relatively common life situations—can increase someone's vitamin needs.

Vitamins are the key to the body's utilization of the food it ingests. Strictly speaking, vitamins don't provide energy or build up the body. Rather, being organic compounds called coenzymes, their prime role is to set the stage for good body performance.

Vitamins don't exist in the body freely; they are liberated from their carbohydrate or protein structures during digestion to be absorbed through the intestine into the bloodstream. General circulation transports them to tissues such as muscle, liver, kidney, and brain. Now they become coenzymes, helping the tissue enzymes convert protein, carbohydrates, and fats into new tissue and new energy. When any of these steps is interfered with—when intake, storage, or vitamin conversion aren't each operating optimally—vitamin deficiency and illness can result.

Few cases of constant, pathological vitamin deficiency exist today in America. But borderline shortages may be more common than we suspect. Food fads, skipped meals, between-meal snacks, munchies, and special diets all take their toll. In addition, smoking greatly reduces vitamin C levels, while alcohol interferes with the use of vitamins B_1, B_6, and folic acid, among others. Fortunately, a large intake of vitamin C supplements is not harmful to the body, although obviously the better solution is to stop smoking. Nor will the vitamin correct damage to the lungs and system. Similarly, in the case of alcohol, although increased vitamin intake is recommended, this won't prevent the development of liver damage. The cycle is classically vicious in instances of alcoholism: Alcohol leads to liver injury, which leads to less vitamin absorption from food, which leads to more intensified liver injury due to unavailable nutrients to repair damaged liver cells.

Unfortunately, vitamin crazes spring up from time to time. A few years back vitamin E was heralded as a modern-day miracle. Not true at all, as proved by the deodorants containing it being banned. Often organic vitamins are hyped as superior to synthetic ones, although evidence that the body can tell the difference is scant. Organic vitamins probably offer no special benefits, yet to many they are more palatable. Documentation does exist proving that badly unbalanced vitamin intake can interfere with proper body functioning. The subject of nutrition deserves a whole book in itself. Indeed, many (perhaps too many, since their conclusions are so contradictory) have already been written. Vitamins are essential to life. But they must be viewed in the overall perspective of nutrition. Seek out the best advice possible before jumping blindly into any self-prescribed vitamin therapy.

If you follow the suggestions of the Food and Drug Administration concerning the recommended daily allowance (U.S. RDA) of the twelve classified vitamins, you can't go far wrong. (U.S. RDA information is

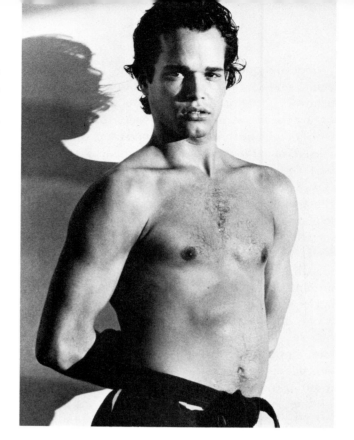

listed on the labels of many food products and vitamin supplements. These tell you what percentage of the U.S. RDA for each nutrient is contained in one serving or dose. Obviously, your daily goal should be 100 percent of the recommendation for each nutrient.)

But if you start popping particular vitamin pills extravagantly, you could be working against your own self-interest. On the other hand, it is conceivable that you do have a special vitamin need that won't be met without taking additional measures. That's why receiving solid advice before popping off the deep end is smart.

RAPID TRANSIT
FASTING

Over the centuries fasting, either as a religious or as a mystical experience or as a foolproof way to lose weight, has undergone waning and waxing acceptance. Improperly practiced, fasting can lead to malnutrition and even starvation. Unfortunately, massive overdoses of vitamins A or D can also disturb the system and likewise prove lethal. *How* a man does anything determines the consequences.

Prolonged fasting should never be undertaken without the supervision of a physician. But if periodic fasting—perhaps one day a week—is pursued regularly and sanely, it shouldn't be detrimental, assuming a man is eating wisely on those days he indulges without overindulging.

Some fasters insist that by avoiding food, they detoxify their systems of pollutants—a dubious notion, since the body is continually ridding itself of waste materials. However, the body can feed itself on its own fat reserves if food isn't supplied, so the value of fasting, from the point of view of looking good, is its sure-fire results in losing weight without resorting to the fads and foibles of other systems. To repeat, though, short, intermittent fastings are acceptable only if a person receives good nutrition when the eating is on. When a man fasts for a day or two, he should drink at least two quarts of water (preferably mineral water) each day. This helps in the "flushing" process and wards off dehydration.

Needless to say, someone in poor health should never fast, even for only twenty-four hours, without first consulting a doctor.

Of course, there are variations on the fasting theme. After a prolonged fast—remember, one should never be undertaken without checking first with your physician—it's usually recommended that you mix a quart of water with a quart of either orange or apricot juice and that you sip teaspoonsfuls throughout the day. On the next day, the fruit juice is drunk undiluted. By the third day, yogurt and an apple may be eaten. Large amounts of water should still be drunk.

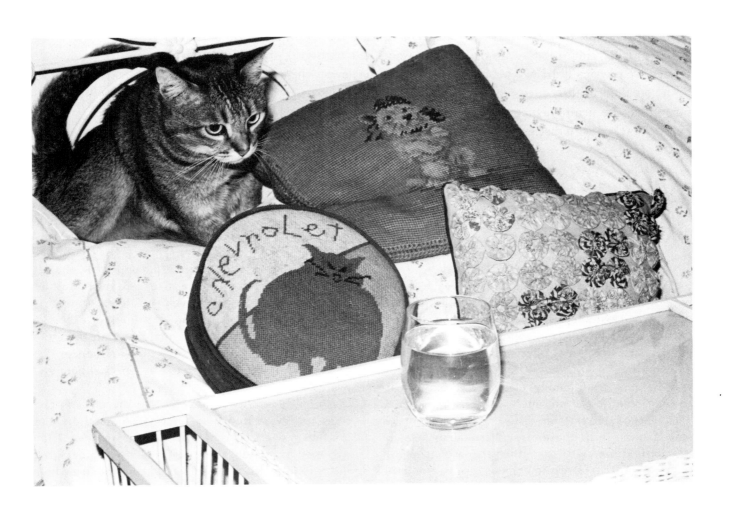

CHAPTER **24**
SHAPING UP
EXERCISE AND TONING

Usually we think of physical fitness in terms of health. Certainly a fit body looks good, and looking good is almost always associated with good health. Men whose bodies are physically fit will probably perform better, even when weakened by illness, than so-called healthy men who have allowed their bodies to go to pot. A sedentary person can be healthy, meaning not ill. But is his body fit? Diagnostically, perhaps he's not racked with disease. Practically, his physical fitness is a mirage.

ON THE MOVE
DAILY DOINGS

Walking and climbing a few stairs may be the extent to which too many modern males use their bodies. A night disco offers other temptations, but dancing at least keeps the body in motion. If you're puffing after one number, you need exercise bad. To get the most from being physical, you should follow a daily routine.

Exercise is traditionally classified into two categories: isometric and isotonic.

Isometric Exercises: Very little or no movement is involved in this form of exercise other than muscle contractions. Primarily to strengthen specific muscles by relying on internal stress to achieve results, isometrics oppose muscle strength against fixed external resis-

tance. This sounds a bit like hitting your head against a brick wall, and it might be so, except head muscles aren't the targets for improvement. Biceps often are. In the initial stages of Indian wrestling, for example, when opponents are equally matched and therefore stalemated, this motionless tension epitomizes the technique of isometric exercise, except that here you exercise alone.

Isotonic Exercises: These involve muscle contractions and extensions that move your joints. Back to the Indian wrestling match: When the stronger of the two men ultimately forces the other's arm back, all the muscles in the arms are stretched through a whole series of movements. Calisthenics, although defined

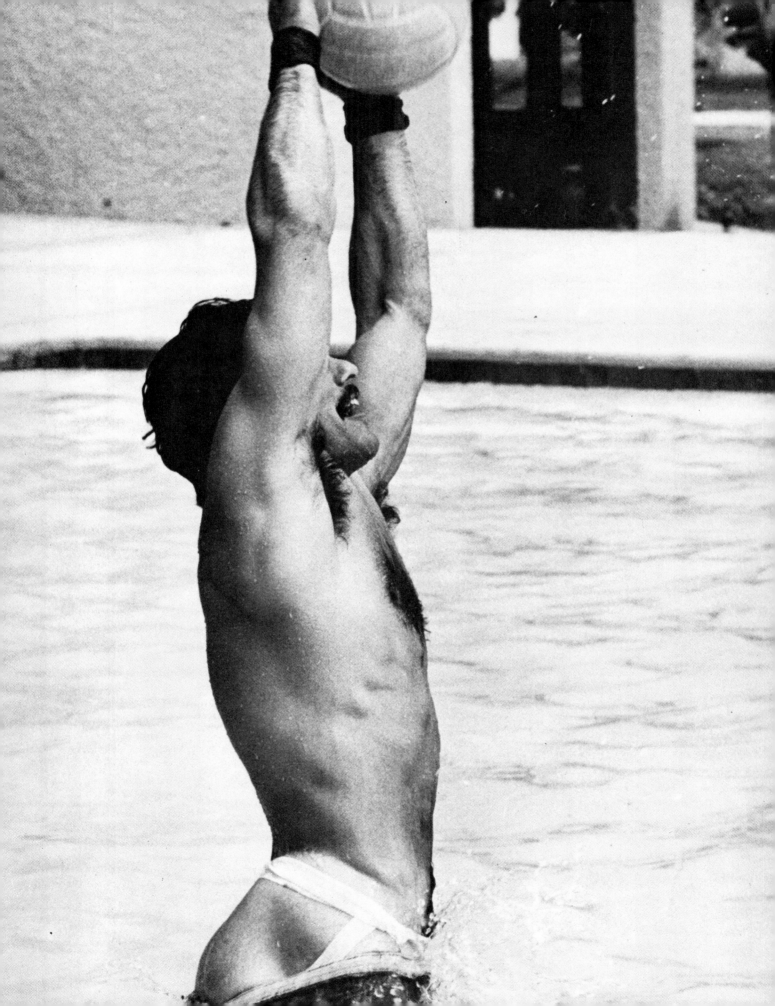

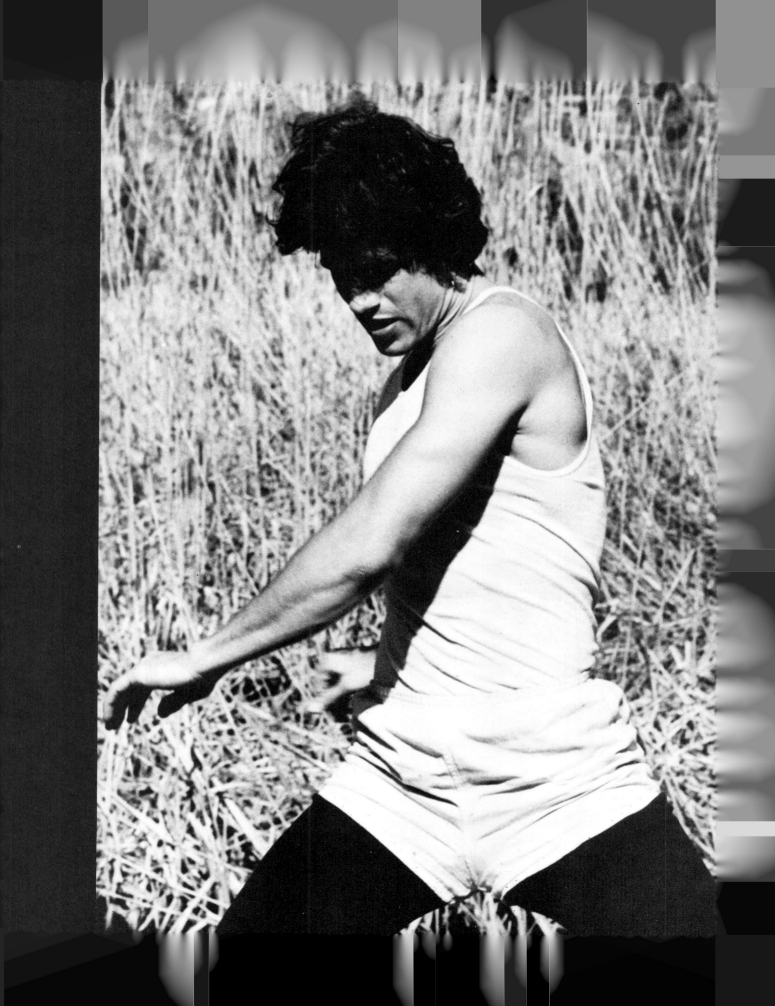

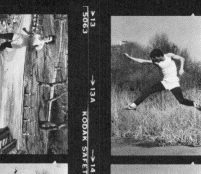
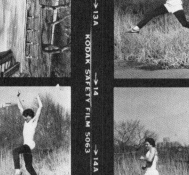
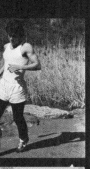
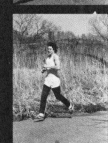
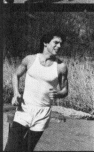
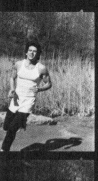
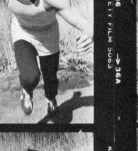
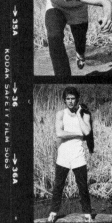
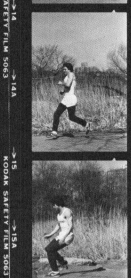
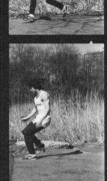
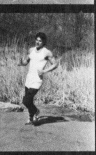
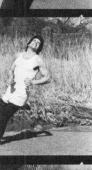
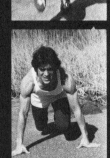
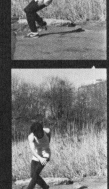
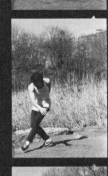
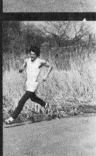
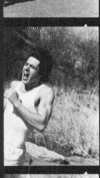
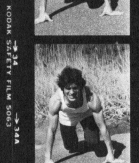
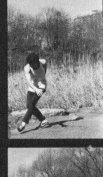
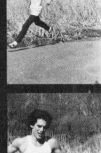
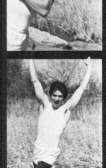
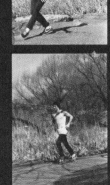
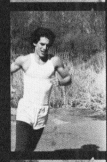
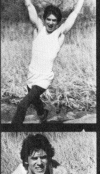
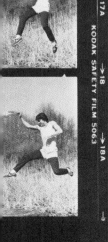
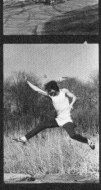
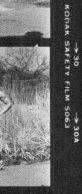
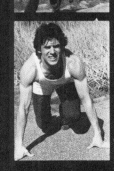

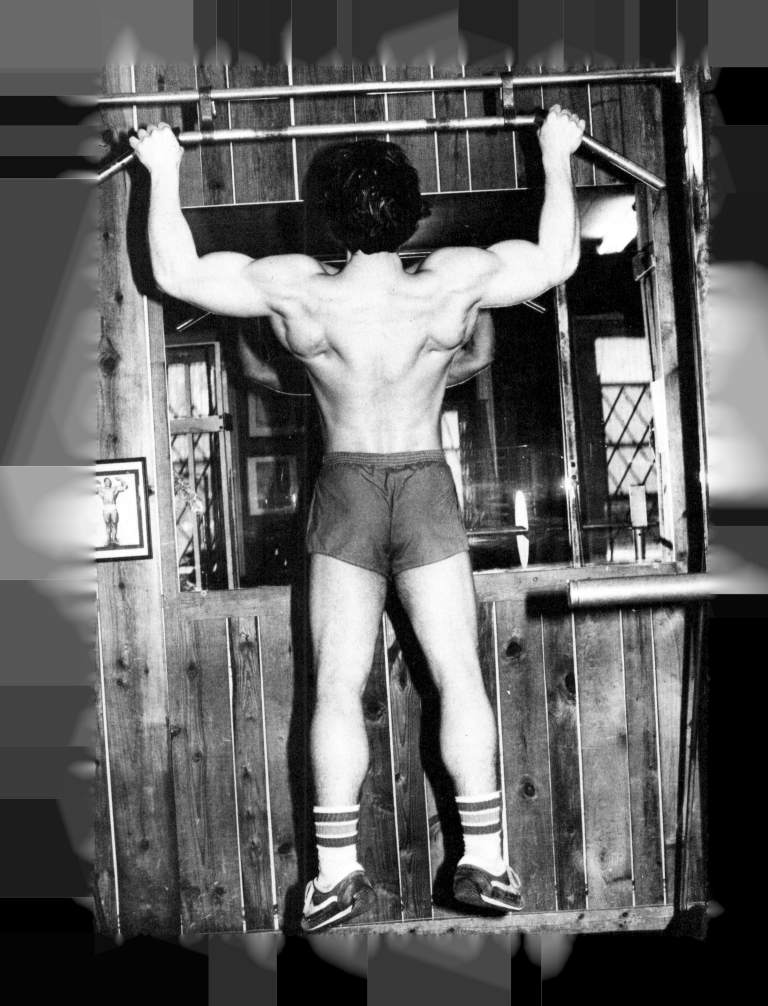

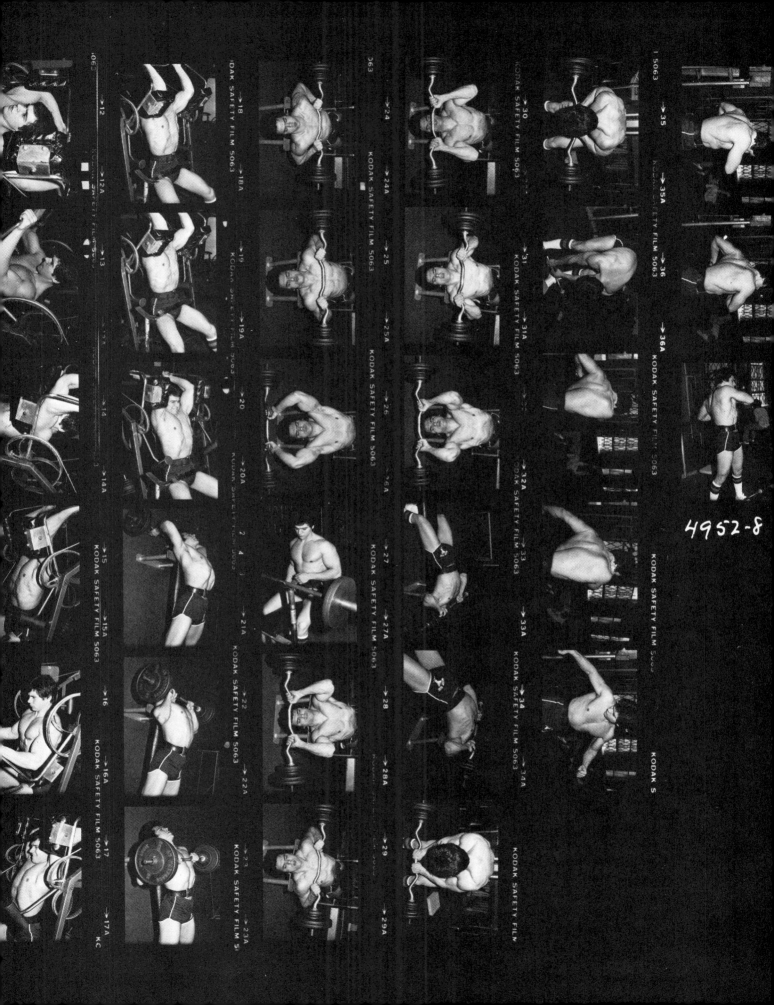

4952-8

as isotonic exercises, cause less muscle strain than weight lifting, which also involves isotonic strength. Both calisthenics and lifting weights build muscle mass; so do isometric exercises, but to a lesser degree. In either type of exercise, overall physical fitness may be sacrificed by concentrating only on localized areas such as the arms or legs. Well-rounded calisthenics, however, tone the entire body.

Another way to classify exercises is according to whether they are anaerobic or aerobic.

Anaerobic Exercises: Anaerobic means "without oxygen." That doesn't mean you hold your breath or stop breathing (although in some cases you may) but that the exercises are of such short duration—like a quick sprint—that oxygen intake is incidental to the activity. Afterward, however, you may have to gulp for air, which is your system's way of ridding any waste products accumulated.

Aerobic Exercises: Surprise! These are "with oxygen." They require endurance and lots of oxygen because they are extended over a length of time. Jogging for an hour is an aerobic exercise. General physical fitness is increased by aerobic exercises, since the cardiovascular and the respiratory systems are strengthened. Anaerobic exercises aren't nearly as helpful in terms of overall body fitness, since they usually exercise only specific muscles. Generally, aerobic exercises are not performed so much to build muscle mass as to tone the body.

Of course, planned physical activity isn't so neatly cut-and-dried as these exercise categories suggest. One's ability to perform an activity without experiencing exhaustion depends upon what the activity is. Someone who has worked out for the purpose of improving his arm muscles might not be able to run around the block without feeling drained, whereas a marathon runner might not be able to press his own weight. Lifting weights is limited by muscular strength. Running depends upon muscular and cardiovascular-respiratory endurance. Yet, in these examples, strength and endurance are separated rather arbitrarily. Good physical fitness programs incorporate goals of both strength and endurance.

Obviously, even if we were all in tip-top shape, our physical abilities would not be the same. Age automatically affects body efficiency. We are confined by the bodies we're born with. Anyone can aspire to being another Samson, but if he's endowed with a five-foot frame, so much for that dream. On the other

hand, one five-foot-no-inch guy can be in better shape than any other five-foot-no-inch fellow alive. But if he's sixty-inches tall and weighs three hundred pounds, he'd better temper his demigod fantasies with patience and common sense. Rushing blindly into strenuous physical exertion is always hazardous to the health, becoming increasingly more dangerous as age and pounds mount. In any instance, the body must be warmed up before partaking in any exercise.

Exhaustion is your body telling you that you've overindulged. You should feel pleasantly tired and relaxed after exercising, but exhilarated shortly thereafter with a sense of well-being, when your body has recomposed itself.

With all the talk about making the body look better, let's not lose sight of the fact that shaping up should make you feel better too. Not only psychologically, because you can stand to gaze at your naked body in a full-length mirror, but also because your mind and body should be relaxed, replenished, ready for anything. Well, just about anything. Physical and mental stress should be alleviated. If an exercise is a drag, then it's not the right exercise. Instead of relaxing yourself, you're probably tensing up. What a waste of time and energy.

BODY WORKS
CHOOSING PHYSICAL ACTIVITY

Exercise programs have become as faddist as diets. Old faithful ones like the Royal Canadian Air Force system are now being challenged by numerous newcomers. Like dieters, exercise disciples are often fickle, quickly interesting themselves in other systems as the current vogue dictates.

Deciding what physical program you should follow is simpler than you realize. Try several and see which one you enjoy the most. No enjoyment, minimal benefits, because your heart won't be in it and you'll probably cheat. Unless a fellow is a catatonic, he should be able to find some activity he likes. Just think of how many there are to choose from. Here is just a partial listing, with a few generalized comments.

Walking Briskly: That's right, just by stepping lively

we can strengthen our hearts and tone our bodies somewhat. Moving at a snail's pace allows the whole system to become lethargic. Needless to say, a jaunty walk won't build your biceps.

Jogging: Naturally, jogging is better than walking since it involves more exertion. But strenuous jogging requires you to be in good condition to begin with. A man over thirty-five should never set off on the jogging trail without first having a "stress check," which can pinpoint silent heart disease. Sudden exercise throws the heart rhythms into a frenzy. Jogging sanely can strengthen the heart, meaning it will pump more blood with less effort. As you become more accustomed to the strain, you can jog with more vigor.

Cycling: This great way to spend a morning or afternoon yields benefits similar to those of jogging, only less of them, unless you're participating in a long-distance race. Any exercise involving sustained, rhythmic, repetitive movements helps the heart; so do deep-breathing exercises. The rigorousness of any physical activity should be increased gradually. Ideally, any exercise program should be performed daily. Practically speaking, three or four times a week may be adequate. Sporadic exercise only puts more strain on the heart sporadically.

Skipping Rope; Rowing: Similar benefits to those of cycling.

Calisthenics: Sit-ups strengthen abdominal muscles. Push-ups work on the torso and upper arms. While affecting muscle masses, calisthenics usually increase muscular strength and endurance as well as size. When various parts of the body are stretched and/or rotated, these areas become more flexible and agile. Naturally, calisthenics consumes body energy, so they, like all calorie-burning exercises, are helpful in losing weight.

Weight Lifting: While increasing physical strength, lifting weights with repetitive pumping motions will also increase muscle size. Seldom is general fitness greatly enhanced.

Dancing: Although male dancers are too often accused of being sissies, their bodies should be more disciplined and in better shape than those of most athletes. A dancer's livelihood depends upon muscular control, not brute power. Dance training includes the best of all exercise programs to achieve endurance and flexibility. On a more practicable basis, performing a waltz may not do a lot for your body, but boogying might. Unless you're a night-crawling regular, the disco doesn't automatically replace the gym. Regularity is a must.

Mechanical Exercise: Many of us are inclined to pass the buck, and concerning exercise, we may shell out bucks in hopes of letting machines do the work for us. Many can't. Electricity-run cycles, for example, which only put somebody through the motions without calling for any physical exertion from the rider, are a pure waste of time and no-energy. Mechanical exercise is helpful only insofar as the body is put into play. Better exercise machines have been developed with graduated goals spelled out in advance, so you truly do have to work to achieve the desired results.

Sex: Fantastic.

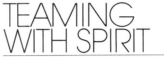

TEAMING WITH SPIRIT
SPORTS AS EXERCISE

Surprisingly, many sports are not as helpful for overall physical fitness as solo activities such as jogging or skipping rope. That's because many opportunities exist in team sports for catching the breath and breaking the rhythms of the activity.

Swimming, whether for personal pleasure or in competition, is the most sustained exercise, since strength, endurance, power, agility, and cardio-vascular-respiratory demands are all high.

Although sports may not be as efficient or effective in shaping you up as more specific exercise programs, they do achieve two extremely beneficial ends: relaxing the body and relaxing the mind. However, win-at-all-cost types tense up their bodies, while tying their emotions in knots. They never receive the full benefits of the sport.

Following are some popular sports, both team and opponent types, with a casual rating on how they score in helping men shape up.

Swimming: As mentioned, it's the best all-around activity for getting and keeping the body in prime shape. Naturally, floating doesn't count. Swimming several laps in a pool daily does.

Skiing: Skiing doesn't build as much physical strength as swimming does, but downhill racing certainly calls for stamina and agility. Muscle masses aren't dramatically increased from the sport, which is fine for many guys who don't want to look like regulars from Muscle Beach.

Tennis: It's in the same league with skiing as far as shaping up goes, although its aid in developing muscular endurance is less. As a visit to any tennis court illustrates, playing tennis doesn't ensure a body beautiful. But imagine how those paunchies would look if they didn't play at all.

Soccer: This increasingly popular sport builds less power than tennis does but more endurance.

Golf: Golf's status as a favorite weekend pastime notwithstanding, as far as shaping up goes, it offers less than nearly all other sports. It does develop heart muscles to some degree. But even canoeing has more to recommend it for general fitness. Maybe the low emphasis on physical demand explains why little old ladies flock to golf courses. (Sorry, Mother.)

Bowling: Worse than golf for what it doesn't do.

Badminton: Not bad at all. It exercises the heart and

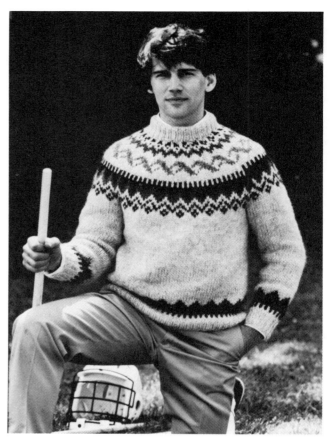

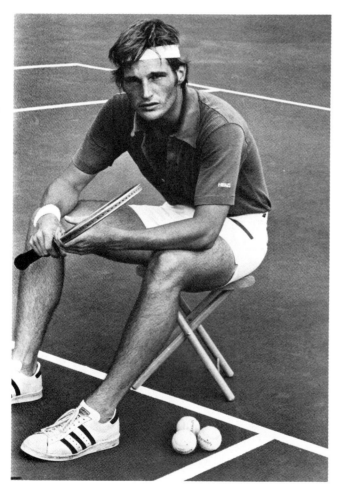

lungs better than baseball while contributing to better coordination.

Handball: Another all-around good activity. Raw strength isn't necessarily increased, but the brisk pace is good for general development.

Hockey: Even though hockey sometimes seems little more than a free-for-all brawl, it does no more for the body than does genteel skating. Both activities develop endurance and agility while taxing (but hopefully not overtaxing) the heart to do its darndest. Muscular strength isn't highly promoted unless the pattern of play brings in boxing elements.

Baseball: It may be the American pastime, but baseball isn't very effective in producing increased strength or agility, though it does improve muscular endurance considerably.

Football: What's Sunday afternoon without the game of the week? Well, if you're sitting and watching it, it does nothing for your body; vicarious activity doesn't tackle inertia. When played, football has the same benefits as baseball, while building more muscular power.

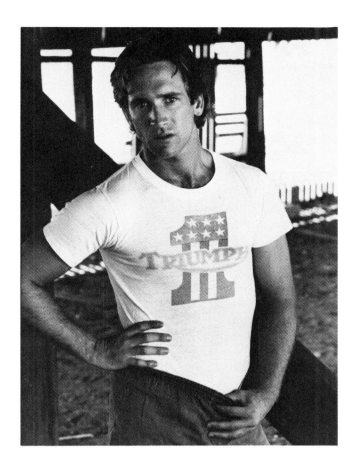

body is being manually manipulated. Many men are afraid to go to a legitimate massage parlor because they don't know where to find one. Too bad, because expert massage is akin to nirvana.

True massage involves stroking and applying pressure to all parts of the body, although different techniques are designated by various names. So-called Swedish, French, and German massages are remarkably similar, although Oriental massage may involve the use of acupuncture and acupressure points. At-home massage, though nice in itself and better as a prelude, is still nothing like the real thing, which involves touching on all muscles in specific, calculated techniques.

The reduction of muscular tension is the major goal of massage, since tight or knotted muscles restrict coordination, agility, and quickness. Blood circulation is stimulated, bringing about a healthier tone to the skin while helping the body to utilize its nutrients

Basketball: Although basketball shouldn't be a rough-and-tumble game, it's a superior one to baseball or football for shaping up since it places more emphasis on developing the cardiovascular-respiratory systems. Musculature won't be influenced a lot, but overall the body will function better.

Water Skiing: It doesn't do a lot for the body—other than helping you receive a first-rate tan—but it's lots of fun.

Sex: Why not repeat it? Often. The nicest team sport around.

MANUAL LABOR
MASSAGE

Some massage parlors actually perform massage. And some masseuses train in physical therapy, not fantasy release. But a certain amount of sensuality is present even in a classic, legal massage, since the

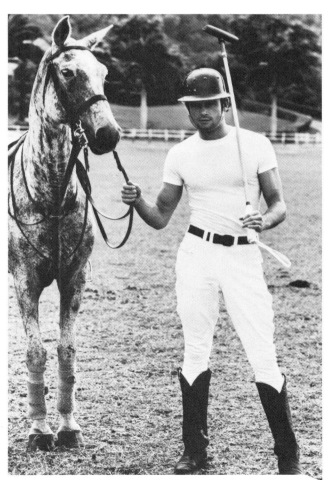

better. Of course, these same benefits are obtained from active exercise but without the psychologically pleasing touch sensations.

Massage after exercise has decided advantages. Waste products are built up during physical exertion, causing chemical changes within the system. Quick movements may have jarred the muscles and joints. Massage soothes the body, helping to reduce soreness and pain (the existence of which would mean that the exercise may have been too strenuous) by activating the circulation. Increased blood flow also helps eliminate toxins from the body.

Massage does not exercise the cardiovascular system as generously as regular exertion, but improved muscle tone can reduce some forms of high blood pressure by strengthening the vein walls.

To repeat, massage won't turn a ninety-pound weakling into Arnold Schwarzenegger, but it can maintain the muscle tone of good, healthy bodies without increasing muscle mass. A body builder who's let himself go can certainly look in worse shape than the fellow who's never lifted any weight greater than that of his own body in the process of climbing onto the masseur's table.

TEMPERATURES RISING
SAUNAS, TURKISH BATHS

Steam rooms are meeting grounds where the body's problems supposedly drip away in a warm atmosphere. Saunas employ dry heat, while most other systems emit wet steam, yet their principles are much the same. By inducing our bodies to sweat, we are presumably ridding them of unnecessary waste, clearing the way for better skin and muscle tone.

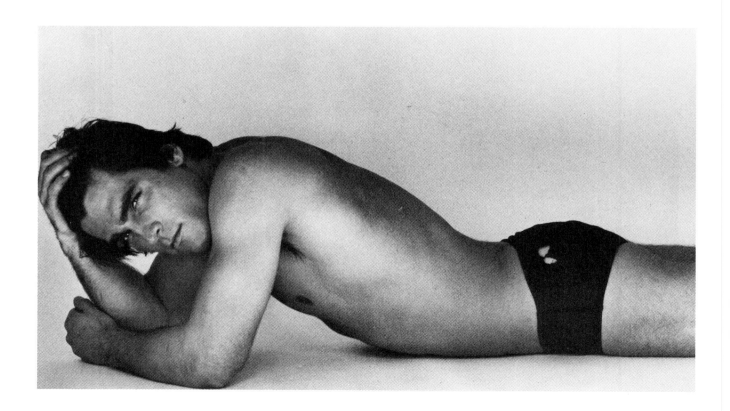

Heat is unquestionably soothing. Applying a heating pad to a sore neck is the perfect proof. However, men with weak hearts are told to play it safe and avoid the hot spots. Saunas and steam rooms may cause too much strain on the ticker, since the high heat dilates the entire vessel network, causing a drop in blood pressure. Then the heart will beat faster, valiantly trying to reassert normalcy by sharply increasing the pulse rate. Even men with healthy hearts may feel tired from the strain on their systems after a sauna or steam treatment. More than half an hour at one sitting is considered unwise; ten minutes is a good limit if done regularly.

Although sweating does detoxify the system somewhat, profuse and prolonged sweating can be dehydrating. Temporary weight loss often results. But as the thirsty body consumes quenching liquid, normal weight is quickly restored. If water isn't taken in, the body remains dehydrated. No good. It's smarter to limit moisture loss in the first place.

Temperatures should not be too hot; above 190 degrees is too much, below 170 degrees insufficient. When subjected to extended and excessive dry heat, nasal membranes may dry out, in turn giving rise to colds, especially if someone steps from a heated environment into a cool draft. Showering after a sauna or steam bath—starting with the water hot and slowly reducing it to cool—prepares the body for external temperature again.

Like massage, the best thing about sweating it out in raised temperatures is the relaxation value. However, since muscles are not manipulated in saunas or steam baths, any toning that results is emphatically secondary, if measurable at all.

Heated pools with whirling waters and a steamy atmosphere are more therapeutic and more toning. Some football players immerse themselves in therapy pools after a particularly rough game. Injured players spend even more time there. However, athletes' lives are hardly passive, so once again relaxation outweighs any reputed toning benefits.

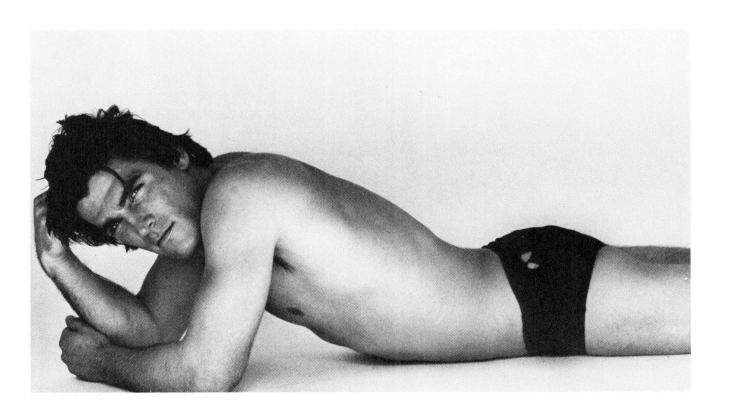

CHAPTER 25
WEATHER VAIN
SEASONAL CONSIDERATIONS

Animals live in seasonal cycles. Not so the human animal, although often he becomes so sedentary in winter that his existence resembles hibernation. Since men don't sprout seasonal fur coats, protection comes from the addition or subtraction of layers of clothing. But the body is always there, covered or uncovered, and seasonal influences affect it.

THE FRIENDLY SKIES
SPRING & FALL

Ah, spring. Ah, fall. The world's in tune. And so should our bodies be. Of course, they're probably not. We've eaten too much during winter, so it's time to shed a few pounds. Or we've caroused during balmy nights and feel drained as much from lack of sleep as from the relentless sun. Shape up we must.

Just as you might want to treat your face to a professional facial come the first inklings of spring and fall, treating your body to a professional massage is an invigorating welcome to the good days ahead.

The friendly seasons are also times to brush away some body detractors. Pumice stones will smooth rough patches on the elbows and knees. Sponges or loofahs help eliminate any coarse cellular buildup on the body. Body rubs with skin conditioners will tone up the muscles for more hiking and sporting around

The friendly skies of spring and fall shine with moderation. Get plenty of rest and relaxation. Work away stress and strain. Use these seasons to build up your resistance for the demands of the rigorous weather ahead.

THE COLD WAR
WINTER

Naturally, it's far better for your body and your system if you don't take an extended winter vacation from exercise. But suspension is better than the life-

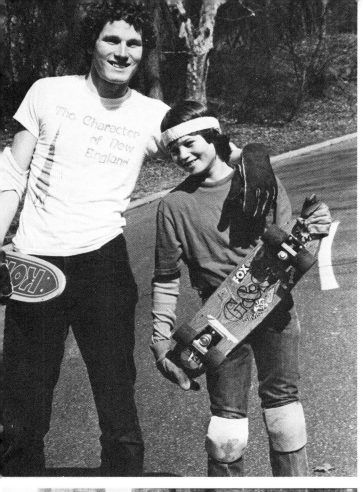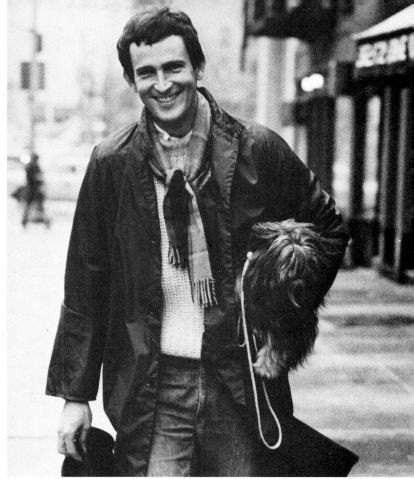
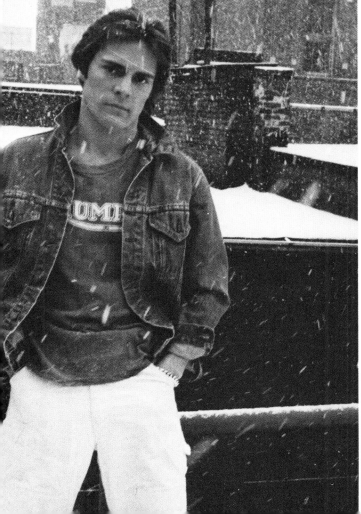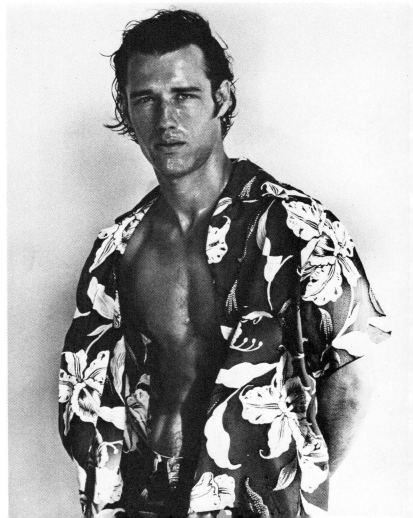

or-death suspense of a coronary. *Never* rush into strenuous exercise in wintry weather without first limbering and warming up the muscles. Work up gradually from easier to more arduous motions. The body should never be traumatized by sudden exertion. Similarly, don't stop suddenly after violent exertion; this too is shocking. But why wreak violence on your body anyway? Sane exercise, particularly during cold spells, is smarter.

If you swim and/or work out at a health club in winter, take extra time to cool off before going outside. Slowly reducing shower heat from hot to cool helps.

Almost all skin experts say that too-frequent bathing is one of the common causes of dry, itchy skin during winter. Showers—not lengthy but just enough to wash the areas of the underarms, feet, and vitals—are the recommended alternative.

Well, even though bathing is supposed to be drying to the skin, it is relaxing and stimulating to the system. Worry warts can massage their bodies with mineral oil before bathing, then wash normally, with or without supplemental bath oils. After bathing and rapidly drying, body lotions will promote moistened, smoother skin. Legs and arms need more attention than the torso. This extra layer of moisturizing protection should help fend off dryness. Body splashes, which contain a fair amount of alcohol to refreshen the skin, shouldn't be doused during intemperate months unless a lubricating lotion or cream is applied over them.

Cold weather inhibits the blood circulation. Fragrance products don't reach their full potential without heat and body warmth to activate them. To get the most bloom, rub extra amounts of cologne on your chest and arms *after* rubbing on a compatible or an unscented protective lotion.

Body massages are relaxing and toning for inactive bodies.

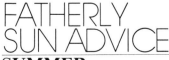

FATHERLY SUN ADVICE
SUMMER

It's no minor coincidence that the first definition in standard dictionaries for tanning is the process of making leather from rawhide. As has been repeated constantly throughout this book, the bronze suntan most people crave changes not only the skin's coloration but its texture as well. It's your own hide you're tanning, and the results can be rawly harmful. Examining the skin mechanisms involved in tanning explains why.

The skin's outer defense is a protein material called keratin, which is thickened by ultraviolet rays. Extra keratin is produced by exposure to the sun and aids in both absorbing and reflecting harmful rays. This thickening doesn't profoundly darken the skin.

"True" tanning is the production of new melanin granules (the yellow/brown pigment) at the base layer of the epidermis. As these pigmented cells and melanin granules migrate closer to the skin's surface, the skin is truly darker from deep down inside. Tanning, then, is caused by the ultraviolet rays of the sun in the burning range. Since a degree of sunburning is a prerequisite to true tanning, any sun preparation that prevents all burning rays from reaching the skin will also keep your tan from being "true." The element of redness (technically called erythema) is not itself all bad except when it's painful. Redness and burn are not synonymous.

Another tanning mechanism of the skin (not considered "true" tanning) is the oxidation by the sun of existing pale melanin that has remained in the skin from a previous tan. It is a simpler and more rapid tan, but you are not as resistant to sunburn.

Although signs of deep tanning may last for months (at least on the body), the major protection against sunburn is not so much the increased melanin (which does help) as the concurrent thickening of the skin (which helps more). The thickening gradually dissipates and offers no protection after approximately two months following the last exposure to the sun.

Atmospheric conditions affect tanning. Sky radiation, which is sunlight scattered in the atmosphere, will produce burning without exposure to direct sunlight. On lightly overcast days, for example, the burning rays are scattered but can still cause severe burning. On the other hand, dirt particles and smoke that pollute urban air may protect you a little against sunburn by absorbing some of the rays. Sunbathing on a rooftop tar beach can be safer than lying under a blanket of clean air, though it doesn't do a lot for your lungs. The higher the altitude, the fewer are the harmful rays that are dispersed. The lower the latitude, the greater the number of burning rays. The hours of

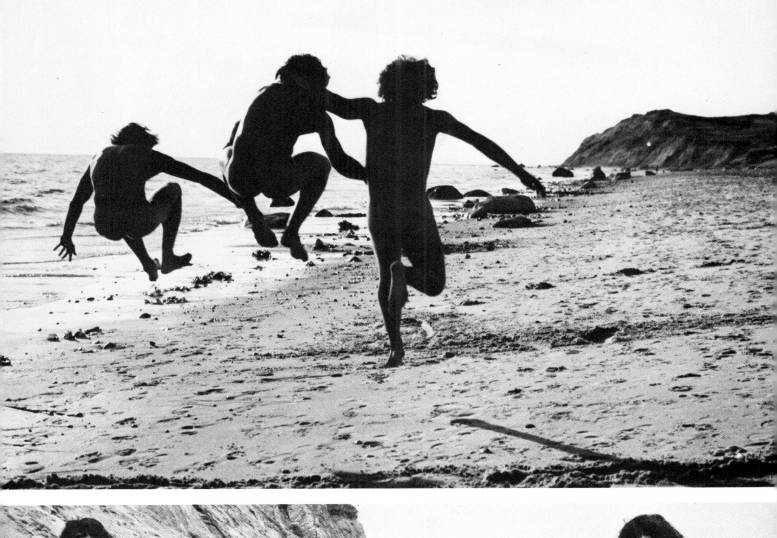

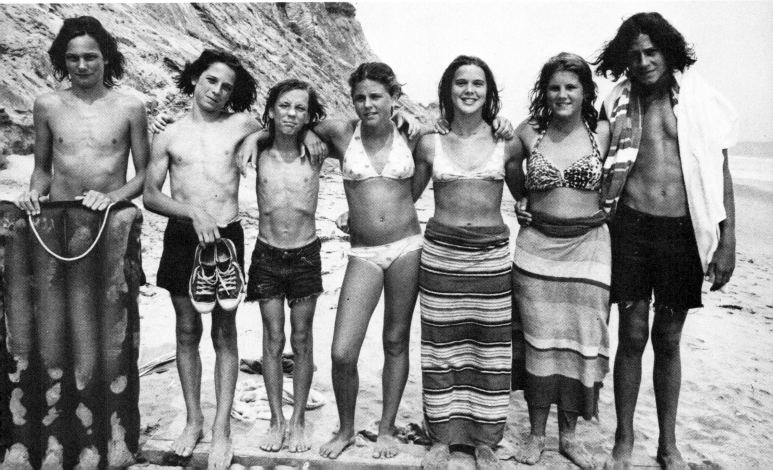

greatest risk are between 10:00 A.M. and 3:00 P.M., with noon's rays their most direct and therefore most potentially dangerous.

On the Beach

Generally, darker skin is less vulnerable to burning. But certain dark-skinned guys burn more easily than blue-eyed blonds. Tanning and burning are individual skin reactions, although oilier skin is more susceptible to burning. The oil tends to "broil" it.

Contrary to what many people think, a sunburn does not convert into a tan; it simply fades away, allowing the tan you acquired to show. Or the skin peels and is more vulnerable to another burn.

Since it takes several hours to twenty-four before the full effects of the sun can be seen on the skin, if you stay on the beach until you turn pleasantly pinkish, you've already gone too far. The only reliable method is to follow a predetermined timetable. The American Medical Association suggests a schedule that seems ridiculously short, but it has proven reliable.

For light-skinned fellows: Initial exposure to sunlight, fifteen minutes; second exposure, twenty; third, thirty; subsequently, based on redness and tenderness. For darker-skinned guys: Begin with twenty minutes and increase the exposure periods by five minutes each day.

However, the recommendation is based on the use of *no* sun products. Even with a lotion, you shouldn't overdo. Start with a maximum of one-hour exposure on the first day, using plenty—more than you think you need—of protective suntan lotion. Increase exposure by a half-hour each day, applying a *bit* less protection each day. Should the skin feel taut or tender, skip the sun for a few days. Remember to moisturize your skin to what seems like excess. It won't be. Unless a product totally blocks out all the ultraviolet rays, your skin can burn at any time, even if you already have a tan.

Several physiological changes occur in the skin when too much light energy is absorbed. Proteins in the tissue become highly excited, retaining energy and heat. The blood vessels dilate, manifested by redness and inflammation.

Usually, if the sunburn is mild, the skin will become pleasingly tanned. To repeat, however: This is not due to the burn turning into a tan but from the redness fading. No way exists to quicken the tanning process during the first days. Your skin will only tan at its natural, predetermined rate, in direct proportion to the amount of sun taken. Too much sun and severe reactions can lead to irregular sloughing of the epidermis, causing sun blotches. Toxic reactions possibly include fever, chill, nausea, delirium, and prostration. Does the hope justify the risk?

Those foregoing are only immediate reactions, occurring within six to twenty-four hours. What else is in store? Wrinkling, thinning and thickening, yellowing, graying, reddening, "liver spots," and scaling possibly at some distant, or not-too-distant, date. Delayed reactions are cumulative and at some point irreversible with each prolonged exposure to the sun.

Each manufacturer of suntan products implies that if its products are used instead of a competitor's or none at all, a "better" or "faster" tan will result. As noted, impossible. Your own skin color and the amount of melanin you produce are the real determinants. The true value of sun preparations is that they either further moisturize the skin or allow you to stay in the sun longer than you otherwise could without burning.

Most suntan preparations contain chemicals that absorb some or all of the burning rays of the sun. Sun *shades* usually refer to opaque barriers, such as zinc oxide, which coat the skin but aren't absorbed into it. They scatter the light so that no rays of any length reach the skin. Sun *blocs* (or *blocks*) may also be opaque types, or they may be liquids, lotions, or oils. When applied, you can't see them. They also eliminate all burning rays. *Sunscreens* vary in the percentage of rays they are capable of deflecting. By law, any suntan preparation claiming to be a deterrent to burning must specifically name the sunscreening chemical on the label. PABA is the most effective shielding agent.

How can you evaluate the oceans of lotions, creams, gels, butters, liquids, and foams that are on the market? With great difficulty. By carefully reading labels, you *should* be able to ascertain which products contain more screens. Underscore the *carefully reading*, too.

To sound tantalizing, some products are called "deep tanning," "dark tanning," and so on. Misleading. Usually these contain less—or no—sunscreens. If a product says "for people who tan easily" or some such jargon, that really means minimal protection. Be careful with these. If you use such preparations thinking you can stay out longer on your first day, you'll be painfully sorry.

Should you burn, there's no quick cure. The burn must run its course. One old-fashioned remedy is to mix sour cream and yoghurt, spreading the mixture over the burn. More up-to-date aids include ointments, wet compresses, and soothing lotions. Or submerging yourself in a cool tub. Wear loose, lightweight clothing. Grin and burn.

About commercial sunburn medications: They contain ingredients intended to reduce pain, but they can cause allergic reactions. If pain is excessive or if blistering is extreme, see a doctor.

For some final words about suntanning, let's clear up a few myths.

The month most propitious for maximum tanning is *not* July. Prime tanning time is June 21 (in the Northern Hemisphere, that is), due to the direct positioning of the sun. Because of the earth's angle of axis, you can get a more severe burn at the end of May than at the beginning of August.

Sitting under an umbrella may *not* protect you from burning. Ultraviolet rays reflect from sand and can even travel through wet, white clothing.

Baby oil mixed with iodine does *not* protect you from the sun. The mixture increases burning risk; the iodine stain eventually washes off.

Spreading extra thick layers of grease or oil on your skin will *not* ensure anything other than the inhibition of normal perspiration, possibly leading to sunstroke.

It is *not* true that you burn more readily on a hazy day. You just become more reckless.

Avoiding the ravages of sunny overindulgence, however, isn't the only dictum for warm-weather grooming. There are potentially many other sun-related problems.

Occasionally, for instance, some colognes will increase the skin's vulnerability to sunlight. A brownish discoloration will often occur where the fragrance has been applied when the skin is exposed to tanning. One commonly used ingredient in citruslike scents, oil of bergamot, is known to photosensitize the skin in this manner. Of course, it's easy to test. Just dab a small amount of any questionable cologne onto an inconspicuous spot, then go out in the sun. If there's no discoloration (and odds are there won't be, since allergic reactions to most fragrances aren't widespread), stop worrying.

A number of skin phenomena are still not truly understood. Polymorphic light eruptions—what most people call rashes—encompass a group of reactions that aren't necessarily allergic, but no one knows all the reasons they occur. Yet it's been shown that during summer, rashes are more likely to occur when sun agents aren't used. A prominent dermatologist always suggests graduating from screens to creams to oils.

Some known allergic sun reactions are related to drugs. Tetracycline, the widely used antibiotic, for example, can produce severe sunburn even with limited use and limited sun exposure. Tranquilizers often cause photoallergic reactions. If you take any drug or medication, check with a doctor or pharmacy about dangers from the sun. Surprisingly, aspirin can help deter sunburn.

For those who don't want to risk sunburn but who want to appear tan, bronzers (see pages 104–108) are fine, but not for the body. So-called quick-tanning lotions that work indoors, without the sun's help, really cause a chemical reaction to stain the skin. Unfortunately, most results look artificial, not to say orange. But applying these quick-tanning lotions, then sunning yourself for half an hour or so, will yield more natural results. Take care, you may still burn if you stay out too long. You might also experience some sun-related reaction to the product that might otherwise have not occurred.

Off the Beach

On the other hand, some skin conditions that are commonly attributed to the sun are not sun related at all.

Tinea versicolor is a fungus infection that's so superficial—no rings or scales, only very, very small, dry, itchy spots on the chest or back—that it may only become visibly noticeable after a person has been in the sun. The infected area won't tan to the same extent as the rest of the skin. A man may mistakenly assume he's reacting abnormally to the sun when it may be a problem he's had for a while.

Vitiligo, a loss of pigmentation indicated by white patches on the skin, is another non-sun-related skin problem that may only become apparent, especially for the fair skinned, after sun exposure. The affected area won't tan at all, so, after sunning, the skin appears mottled.

Many skin problems, however, are heavily influ-

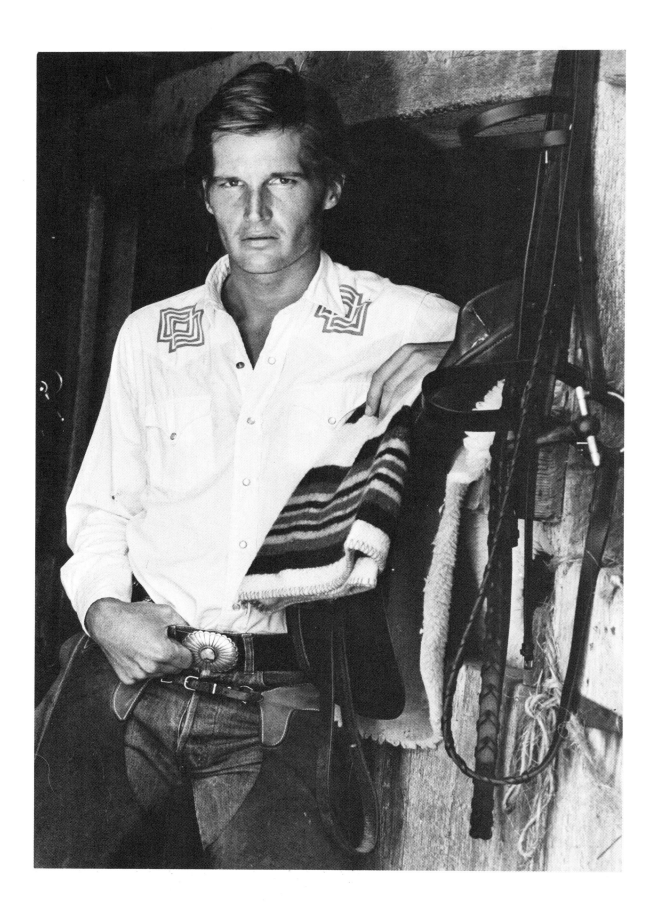

enced, if not by the sun exclusively, at least by the side effects of the summer life-style. *Intertrigo*—hell, you know it as jock itch—is definitely more prevalent during summer. Caused by the combination of heat, perspiration, and maceration of the skin, it's a yeast/fungus infection that causes the skin to become very raw. Compounding this private problem can be an allergic reaction some men have to elastic in swimsuits and underwear. The best defense is to hang loose.

Miliaria, another form of heat rash, produces an inflammation of the sweat glands. Sometimes called prickly heat, it's characterized by redness and burning. If someone perspires excessively and the perspiration gets trapped under the skin, the sweat ducts will get clogged. Perspiration can't escape, so there's breakage *under* the skin, causing an irritation.

Following such rashes the skin can become further irritated, particularly by scratching and macerating the skin; then *impetigo,* a contagious infection, can occur.

To avoid the heat/sweat/rash syndrome, stay dry and cool. That's obviously hard to do on the beach, but you should towel dry as carefully and thoroughly as possible. Don't sit around in a wet bathing suit or ripe sneakers. When out of the sun, talcum powder is cooling. And should rashes appear, stay extra cool indoors, preferably in an air-conditioned place. Don't wear tight or binding clothes. If the rash isn't gone within a week, see a physician.

Paradoxically, although many people think otherwise, summer skin problems are seldom related to uncleanliness. Conversely, some believe overcleansing can dry the skin. Strange, but the effects of chapping—which is really what overly dry skin becomes—can be produced clinically during winter, but it's virtually impossible to do so during the summer. Drying from overcleansing is solely a winter problem.

Extra baths and showers, then, may not be a deterrent to potential skin problems, but they can't hurt, either.

Of course, that problem of dry skin from the sun, if not from bathing, still exists. Body lotions should be spread everywhere the sun touches. Nude sun idolators, that means *everywhere.*

Summer heat causes increased perspiration, hence more difficulty controlling odor. Yet, reportedly bathing with deodorant soaps increases the likelihood of sunburn. Maybe you'll have to use two body soaps after all, an antibacterial/deodorant type for the guilty areas, plus another brand for the rest of the body.

Although swimming is a terrific exercise for the body, lengthy laps in the pool or frolics in the waves both work to dehydrate the skin. The remedy? Another plunge into water, but this time into a cooling bath with bath oils to replenish the moisture loss. This is a good idea even if you don't go near the water.

Most of us want to cut a good figure in bathing suits. Diet mania strikes. Don't go crazy; eat lightly but well. Take vitamin supplements.

Since heat makes colognes more intense on the body, summer calls for a light touch.

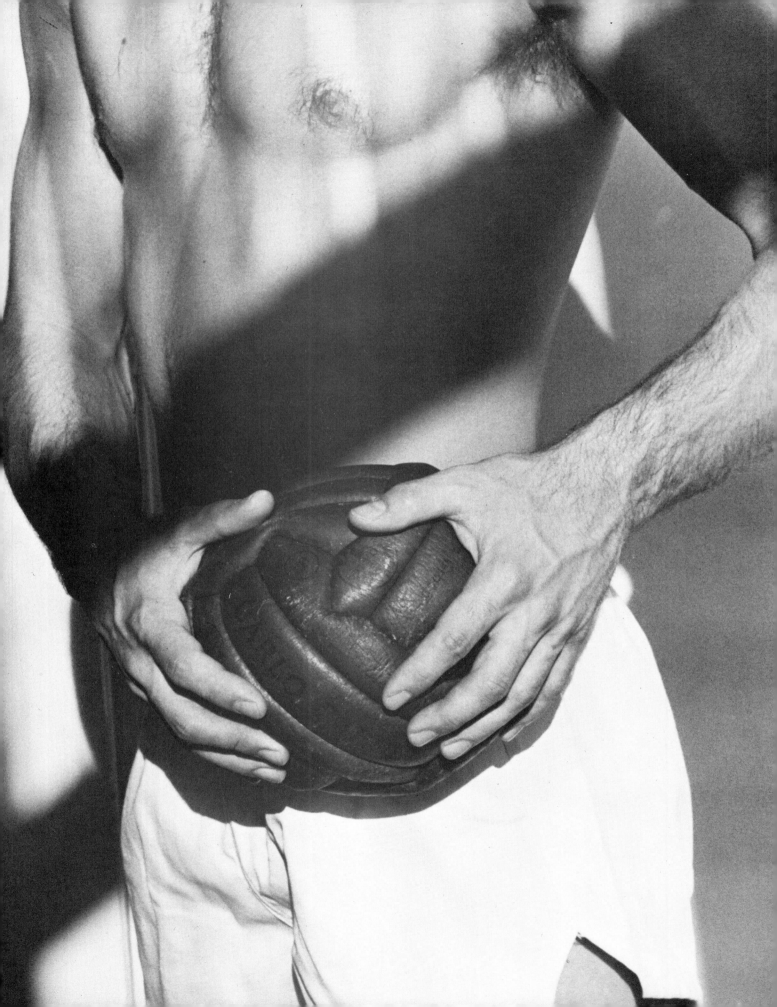

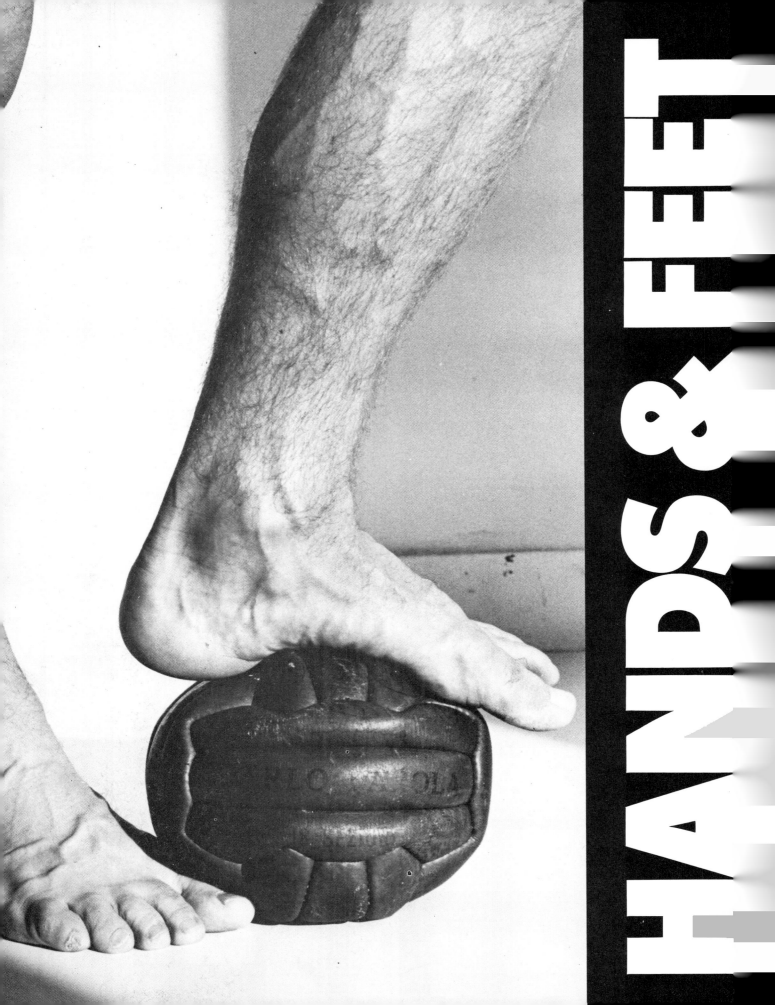

HANDS & FEET

CHAPTER 26

GETTING CLIPPED
NAIL CARE

Some females claim that they find men's hands and bare feet terribly sexy. A rather bizarre preoccupation. Of course, maybe these women are fetishists in disguise and travel in specialized circles. Nonetheless, good grooming should focus some attention on these oft-ignored, nonglamorous appendages. Nail care is the logical beginning.

DIGITAL WATCH
AT-HOME MANICURES & PEDICURES

Since what we see of our skin and hair is already dead, why should fingernails and toenails be any different? Yup, they're nonliving too. Trimming and filing can't hurt, so nail care needn't seem like a trip to the dentist.

Although manicures and pedicures sound terribly elitist, both procedures are easily performed at home and offer a hefty lift to the appearance, though not necessarily to one's sex life. Ragged, dirty nails on a man suggest overall uncleanliness and a lack of self-respect.

Manicures

Many fellows are content to use the key-chain variety of nail clippers. Well, they clip, they dig, they file, but without finesse. Giving oneself a semiprofessional manicure takes only several more minutes but has far superior results.

Necessary equipment includes curved nail scissors; an emery board (or a more costly, diamond-dusted metal file—the dime-store types are too harsh and can cause breakage); a bowl of lukewarm, soapy water (yes, mild liquid dishwashing detergents are acceptable); orange sticks (or Q-tips); a pumice stone; and a hand lotion or cream. Optional: A nail brush, cuticle cream or conditioner (or petroleum jelly), and a nail buffer.

1

First wash and dry the hands. If the nails are longish, trim them with the nail scissors to the desired length and shape. Most men prefer short nails that conform

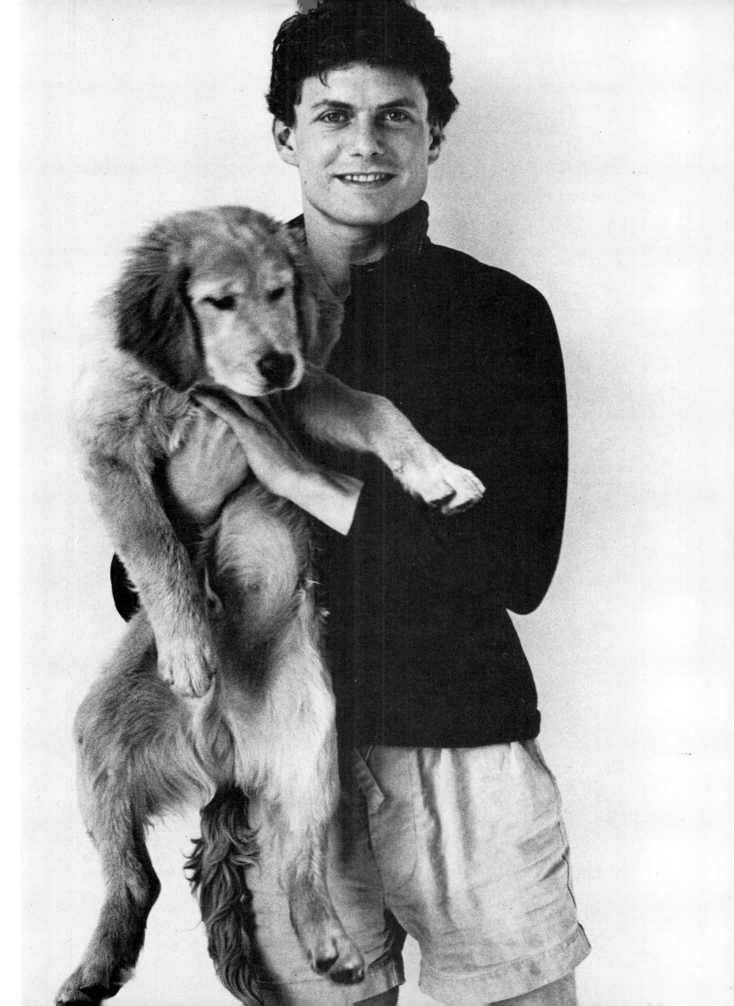

to the curve of the fingertip. Ovals or points are *de trop*. Either side of the nail should be curved, since squared and sharp edges near the tender fingertips invite hangnails.

2

After the initial trimming, smooth the clipped nails with an emery board by filing from the sides to the center at about a 45-degree angle on the underside of the nail.

3

Soak the fingertips in the bowl of sudsy water for two minutes, thereby both cleansing the nails and softening the cuticles, those strips of hardened skin at the base of the fingernails (and toenails, too).

3A

To ensure thorough cleansing of the nails, some manicurists recommend scrubbing the surfaces with a nail brush at this point. The scrubbing may be unnecessary, but it's harmless unless nails are extremely weak. Decide for yourself; using a nail brush is optional.

4

If the cuticles are toughly resistant, rub a small amount of cuticle cream or petroleum jelly into them. If they're sufficiently softened by the soaking, don't bother. *Gently* push back the cuticles with an orange stick tipped with sterile cotton. (A Q-tip will also do.) Fingernail growth is controlled in the "half moon" area at the base of the nail. If the cuticle is injured or this part of the nail is treated too roughly, the growing nail will emerge spotty.

5

When the cuticle is abused and ragged, it should be *carefully* clipped but not totally removed with the curved scissors. The cuticle isn't snaggly? Leave well enough alone. Either way, if any nails are pushing into their surrounding skin (the precursor to hangnails), clip the offending protuberances with nail scissors so they don't.

6

Sweeping the pumice stone lightly, whisk away any dead skin around the nails. Now is also a good time to rub away nicotine stains and assorted uglies that may cling to the fingers. Remember, though, it's skin you're sanding, not wood.

7

Soak the fingers again in the soapy solution for thirty seconds or so to dislodge any foreign particles.

8

Remove the fingers, rinse, and dry. Smooth on a small amount of hand lotion or cream to soothe the skin. Rub a little into the cuticles to keep them soft. (Massaging a dollop of hand lotion into the cuticles during every application of hand lotion, then easily pushing back the cuticles, keeps them amenable for the next manicure.)

9

Buffing the nails with a chamois buffer imparts a healthy, shiny gloss. A matter of personal taste, this step is also optional. So is the application of a colorless coat of polish termed a name glaze.

Surprisingly, although cutting the hair doesn't make it grow any faster or slower, clipping the nails promotes accelerated regrowth. That doesn't mean nail care is best if only a sometime thing. Since nails contact as much dirt as hands, weekly at-home manicures are highly recommended. A few nightly brushes with an emery board can't hurt. Needless to say, biting nails is a no-no.

Pedicures

Pedicures are more cumbersome to self-administer than manicures. For one thing, feet won't fit into that little bowl of soapy water. Cooperatively, toenails grow more slowly than fingernails.

The steps in a pedicure are much the same as for a manicure, except the initial clipping of the nails shouldn't end with curves. To prevent ingrown nails, the toenails should be clipped squarely, straight

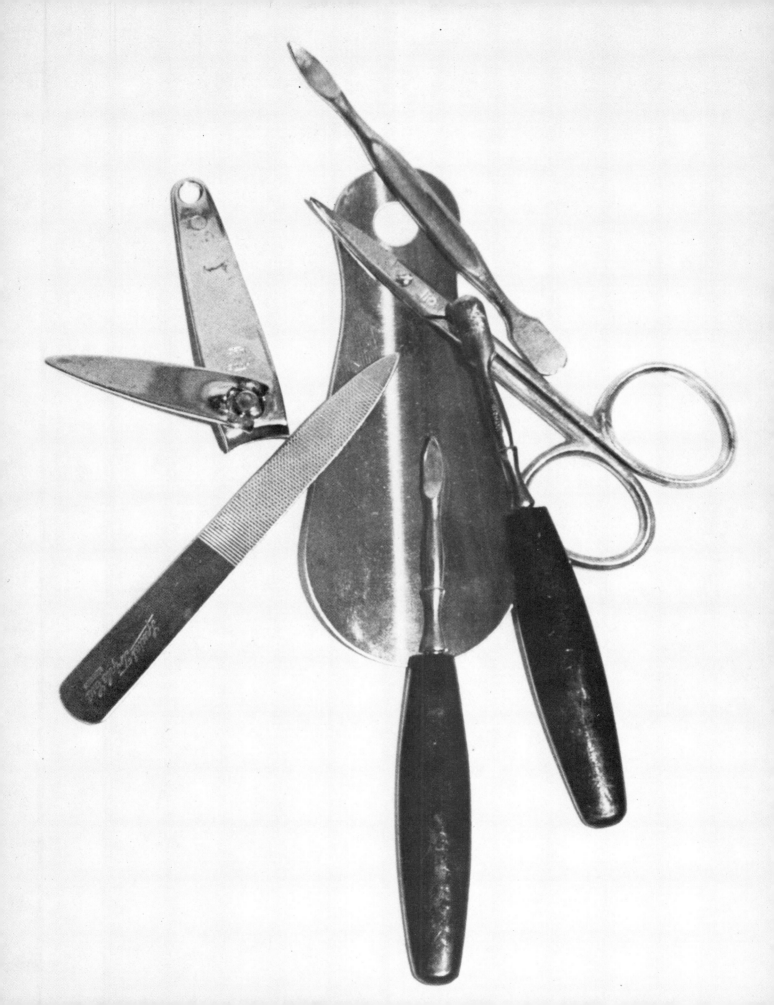

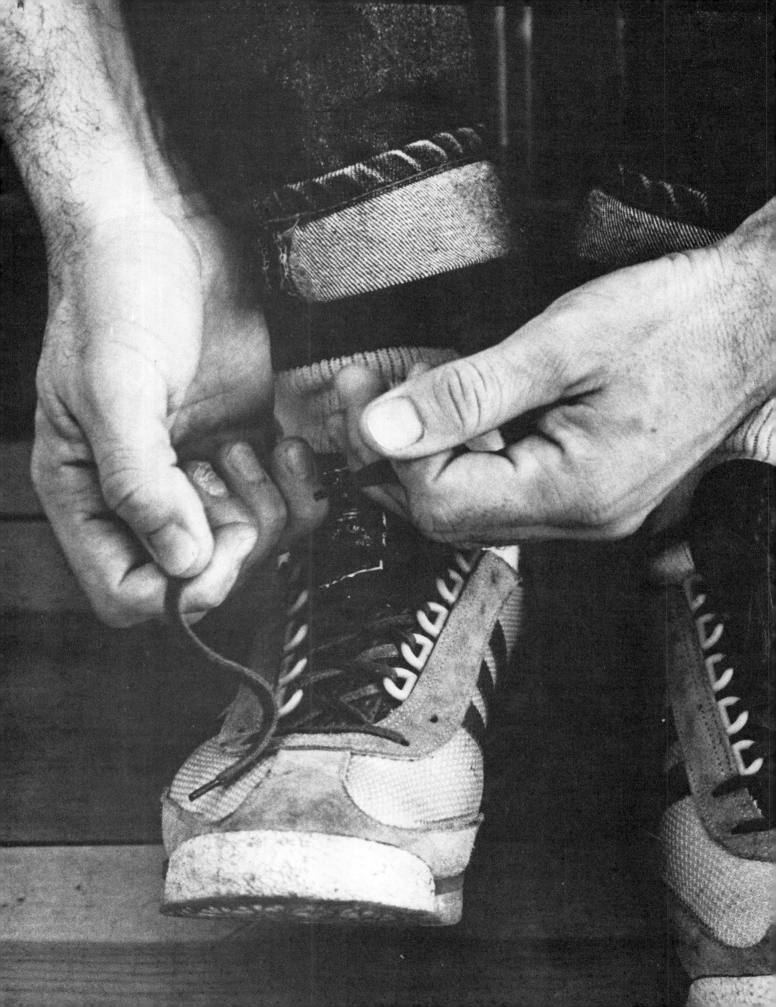

across. Not too short, or the square edges may pierce the skin and produce ingrown nails anyway. The big toe is the most vulnerable. Toenail clippers, with their extra leverage and straight cutting edges, do a better and easier job than curved fingernail scissors.

Since sore feet enjoy it so much, why not extend the soaking period from two to at least ten or fifteen minutes? Purely relaxing, this also increases circulation. Soaking in foot salts instead of soap helps soften the skin even more and combats odor at the same time.

After soaking, push back the cuticles. These seldom, if ever, need any trimming. Now use the pumice stone to remove dead skin. If you have calluses or corns, you shouldn't have. Almost invariably the consequence of ill-fitting shoes, both are the result of prolonged pressure and friction. The body produces these unsightly little devils to protect itself from the aggravating circumstance. So, first remove the cause and then worry about removing the effect. Otherwise, eliminating the calluses and/or corns will only be temporary anyway. Superficially much alike, both corns and calluses are pronounced skin thickenings on the feet, usually the result of constant rubbing over bony areas. However, corns have a regular round shape and a core, while calluses do not. However, they never arise without a warning: Your feet ache and your toes hurt. If you have either affliction, what are you, a masochist?

Enough lecturing. To the practical matter of ridding these thickened skin areas: You can't remove corns. Or at least you shouldn't. Cone-shaped, they may extend as far beneath the surface as to the joint of the toe. This extreme situation eventually leads to painful bursitis. For heaven's sake, don't use a razor blade to cut them away. The job probably won't be complete and the risk is horrendous. With corns, see a physician.

So-called soft corns, usually found between the toes rather than on the tops of them, are soft because of the moisture from perspiration. White and soggy, soft corns are self-treated by drying with rubbing alcohol and putting some lamb's wool between the adjoining toes. Then they may or may not go away. If not, see a doctor. Infections that sometimes accompany soft corns always require medical attention.

Calluses, on the other hand, can be self-removed with extreme care if not too advanced. Most often located above bony areas or on the fleshy part of the foot called the plantar pad, calluses can be pumiced away after soaking. If too deep and thick (meaning cutting is necessary), the removal should only be executed by a physician. Feet do arduous work supporting the entire weight of the body. They shouldn't be treated lightly or haphazardly.

After using the pumice stone to rid cellular buildup and to remove rough skin patches from the feet, the at-home pedicure winds up with massaging a sparse amount of lotion, perhaps the same hand lotion or cream that completes the manicure, over the entire foot. Soothing to the feet, the emollients also help smooth the rough skin on the heels. But feet should never be too moist, since moisture invites the breeding of bacteria. After applying the lotion, dousing the feet with foot powder or talc, then rubbing it between all the toes, will keep the feet drier longer.

Buffing the toenails is gilding the lily. Well, gilding the dandelion.

NAIL SAFE
PROFESSIONAL MANICURES & PEDICURES

Although nail care can be self-performed adequately, it's easier—and more self-indulgent—if done by a professional for luxury's sake from time to time. Many otherwise intrepid men are timid about receiving manicures and pedicures, possibly because they think the nails will be polished. It's true that some professionals conclude the job with a clear polish, but a guy can always shout an emphatic "No!" at this stage. Freedom reigns.

Manicures

The at-home steps are embellished, possibly out of showmanship, by the professional manicurist, who will most likely wield some specialized tools as well. Representative of manicures as given in salons is the following step-by-step description.

1

The nails are first cut and shaped with curved nail scissors.

2

The nail edges are lightly filed and smoothed with an emery board. Metal files, unless they are diamond-dusted, are almost never used by professionals.

3

Cleaning beneath the nail is done with a slender stick tipped with cotton. (Note: This step is usually eliminated at home on the premise that initial hand washing removes most dirt from beneath nails. Soaking, which comes later, should remove any dirt that might still be there.)

4

The emery board is used again. Why is hard to fathom, but if the manicurists' hands are soft, who complains?

5

The fingers are now soaked in warm, sudsy water to further cleanse the nails and to soften the cuticles. After removal from the solution, some manicurists use a nail brush to augment the cleaning. (It is to be hoped that most men's nails are not *that* filthy.)

6

Cuticle oil or cream is massaged into the cuticles, which are then pushed back. Many professionals use a so-called cuticle knife, the edge of which is sharpened to lift as well as push. Extreme care is taken to be gentle.

7

Often, though not always, professionals will nip away some but not all of the cuticle with specially designed scissors. This does give a more streamlined appearance to the fingernails, but it also prompts the cuticles to grow faster. It's reasonable for a man to

ask a manicurist not to clip the cuticles unless they are ragged.

8

Hangnails, if any, are also removed with the cuticle scissors.

9

Now comes the nifty part. A lotion is massaged into the wrists and hands to relax and soothe the muscles. Supposedly this stimulates circulation, which in turn stimulates nail growth. A thoroughly shaky premise but a thoroughly enjoyable experience.

10

The nails are wiped clean with cotton balls so that another moisturizing cream can be applied.

11

This cream is polished to a discreet shine, usually with the aid of a chamois buffer.

12

If desired, a clear polish to strengthen and protect the nails may be applied. Most men forego this step.

13

The manicurist may rub a white pencil beneath the nails to delineate the natural white more sharply.

14

The neatly nailed man pays the receptionist for the service, adding a hefty tip for the manicurist. Giving less than 20 percent is miserly.

Pedicures

A professional pedicure is likewise an extended and expanded version of the at-home procedure. Instead of simply soaking the feet in an oversized bowl, a man may plunge his feet into a water-vibrating machine. Just for kicks, the pedicurist may separate his toes with cute little paper pompoms when performing the various clippings, trimmings, and filings. Rough spots and calluses may be removed not by a pumice stone but rather by implements that look strangely like little cheese slicers. Only a demented pedicurist will sk a male if he wants toenail polish.

CHAPTER 27

ARCH DE TRIOMPHE
FOOT CARE

Li'l Abner wasn't the shnook that his nemesis Evil Eye Fleagle hoped. After all, any guy who runs around barefoot can't be all that dumb: It's one sure way to keep the feet healthy, if not wealthy, and it's a wise way to fend off foot odor besides. Feet aren't exactly way up there on a pedestal, but maybe they should be. They constantly and literally keep us from falling flat on our noses. Foot care is no pedestrian matter.

FIRM FOOTING
DAILY CONSIDERATIONS

Most foot problems stem from ill-fitting shoes that cramp the toes or don't offer enough support. Before even contemplating any other factors, if your shoes are uncomfortable, rush out and spring for new ones that feel good.

Bad posture also contributes to tired, sore feet. Keep yourself in a good upright position and your feet will walk happy, provided, of course, those Italian pointed shoes don't pinch the piggies.

As with all other body areas, foot grooming begins with proper cleansing. Since the feet are so populous with oil-producing glands, they demand extra efforts. Inside shoes are heat and moisture, germs, and decaying matter. Warm moisture keeps the pores of the feet pumping, creating a perfect breeding place for bac-

teria, which not only cause foot odor but present a welcome mat to infection as well. Consequently, feet should be cleansed at least twice a day. (Are those bellows of disbelief? Calm yourself. No one is pointing a pistol at your head and commanding you to do so out of fear for your life. You *should* wash your feet twice daily, but what sane man does unless he's been working in the fields or working out at the gym? Be a little indulgent. Read the following as an ideal regimen. Then go about doing whatever you choose. That's the whole idea of this book: to give you the rationale for why certain procedures should be followed, but leaving the choices entirely in your own hands, where they rightly belong.)

Most men cleanse their feet while bathing or show-

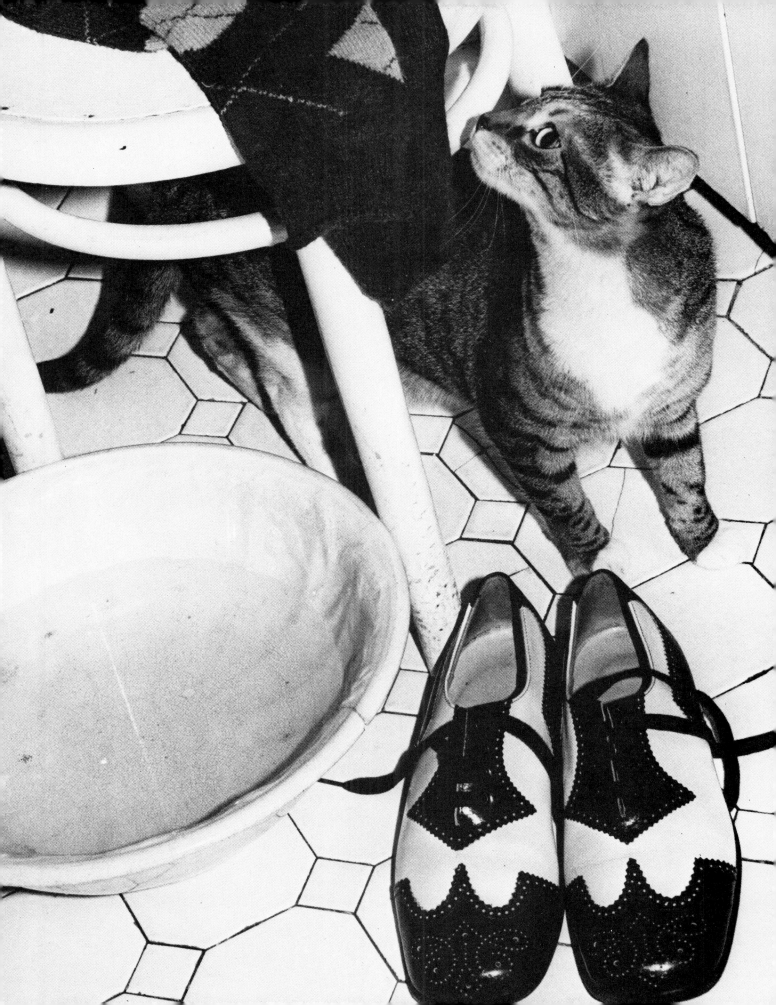

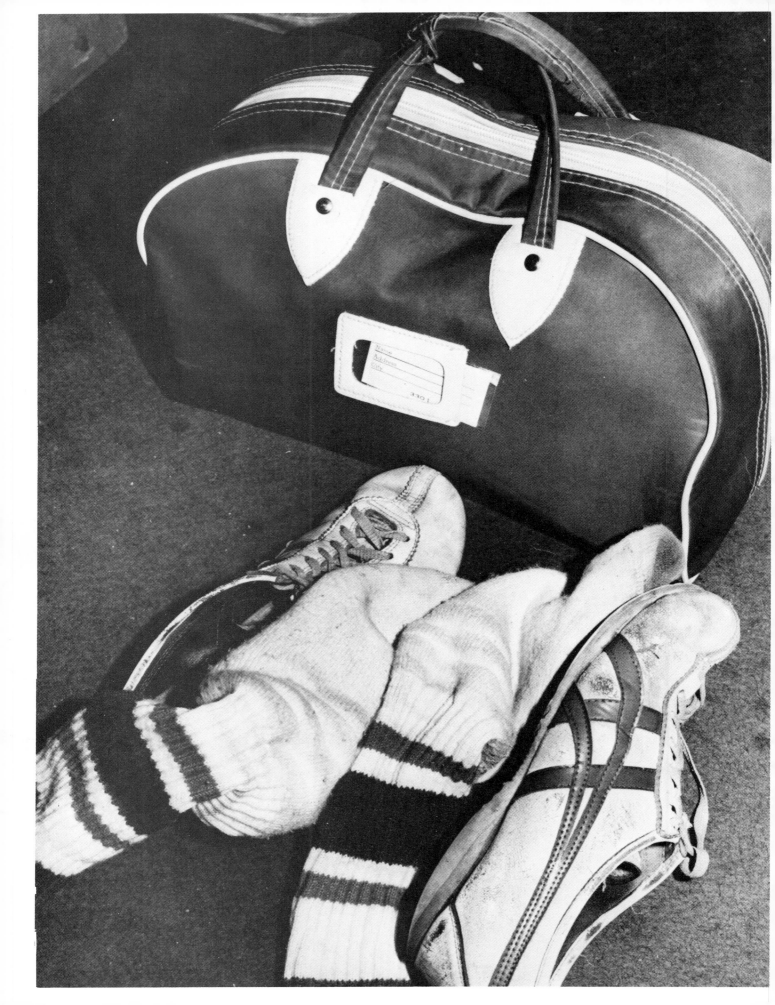

ering. Acceptable but incomplete. A better regimen is to wash them with warm water and soap, rinse with cold water, then dry carefully. Sprinkle the feet with alcohol, making sure you spread your toes, so the skin between them is well doused. After waiting a few seconds, towel away any moisture that hasn't evaporated. (While this technique is always helpful, doing it after swimming or showering in a public place fights common communicable foot diseases.) Once the feet are thoroughly and absolutely dry, douse with some foot powder. Body talcs can suffice in a pinch, but foot powders are heavier in texture, thus more absorbent. Also, they usually have more antibacterial ingredients. Follow this routine every morning. (If you experience particularly troublesome foot odor, you may want to use a foot deodorant spray as well. If so, apply it after the alcohol treatment and allow it to dry before adding the powder.)

In the evening, soak your feet in foot bath salts dissolved in hot water. If your feet are consistently happy, plain hot water will do. Soaking stimulates the local blood supply and promotes circulation, both of which bring relaxation. Relief, too, if needed. In addition, soaking softens the rough outer layer of the skin (more so with the addition of bath salts), while removing dirt or accumulated oils. Dry the feet carefully. (Odds are you'll only do this once a week, if at all, but you'd be surprised how good it feels.)

Now is the ideal time to massage your feet. Nothing works better than the hands, preferably someone else's. If you must go it alone, massage your feet in the following manner, first one foot, then the other.

Start by kneading the sole with your fist. Next, holding your feet between both hands, first give a circular thumb massage to the top, then the bottom. Follow this with a fingertip rubbing of the ankle. Now, still using your fingertips, apply pressure to the heel. Run your thumb along each tendon in the top of the foot while squeezing the foot with hard pumping actions three times between your hands. A twisting massage of each toe is the final step.

Now it's clear why it's preferable that someone else gives the massage, isn't it? All that stretching to reach and hold the feet isn't duck soup. Vibrators aren't as effective, but they do a decent job and are undeniably easier to use than your own fingers.

After massaging, apply a light moisturizer to your feet to keep them soft. Blot away excess between the toes with a tissue. Use a foot powder if you like.

Feet should also be exercised daily to strengthen them. (Stop cackling.) If you'll exercise them only now and again, skip it, since irregular and brief efforts yield zip. Picking up marbles with your toes strengthens them and your arches. (You can substitute wads of paper or pencils if you've lost all your marbles.) A good time to exercise feet is before the evening—or whenever, if ever—soak, since you'll probably dirty your bare feet. Speaking of which. Walking barefoot on a firm surface is another good exercise.

Feet need ventilation not only to ward off foot odor, but also to breathe. Sandals not only look good but they also air the feet. Temperatures permitting.

Athlete's foot doesn't only afflict sportsmen. It can be a fungal infection or caused by various types of bacteria. Whenever the feet are warm and moist—which they can often be during the summer—all types of fungi are in their milieu. Stopping athlete's foot depends upon scrupulous hygiene. Keep the feet dry, dry, dry. Wipe them carefully between the toes, always removing moist debris there. Don't wear heavy socks that prime feet for sweating unless you need them for a particular sport. Even then, put them on just before playing, take them off immediately after and air the feet until you can wash them.

Should athlete's foot strike, try one of the over-the-counter remedies. Ubiquitous powders are best sprinkled inside socks and shoes. Easier to apply and more thorough are liquid preparations.

Don't let the infection get out of hand. Left unattended, athlete's foot can spread to the soles and under the toenails. Then getting the disease under control is next to impossible. Similar types of infection can affect the hands and fingernails. They are no less serious. If self-prescribed medications don't clear up the situation within a week, get thyself to a physician for healing.

If you're reading this book erratically, go back to Chapter 28, "Getting Clipped: Nail Care." Do not collect two hundred dollars.

LA GRIP
HAND CARE

It doesn't take Sherlockian powers to observe that hand care gets right down to the nitty gritty of good grooming. Any armchair detective knows that hands are good gauges for deducing age. If you want to throw these bloodhounds off the scent, try treating your hands more kindly. Manicures, of course, should be an integral part of your routine; see Chapter 26, "Getting Clipped: Nail Care." After all, your hands do a lot for you; why not do something for them?

VELVET-GLOVE TREATMENT
DAILY CONSIDERATIONS

Hands can never be too clean, but they can be harshly cleansed too often. Most hand soaps are not the mildest, on the premise that hands do a lot of dirty work. But washing hands à la Lady Macbeth is not only compulsive behavior, it's overly drying. During every cleansing, any natural protection that the skin possesses is washed away. On the palms, this isn't very serious, for they are amply supplied with oil glands, but the tops of the hands can become dehydrated, rough, and red. Since it obviously isn't practical to moisturize whenever you wash them, it's doubly important to do a good job when you do. Yes, use a hand cream every night and every morning. So-called

housewives' hands aren't confined to those who do dishes. Actually, this skin irritation results from extended contact with detergents and other chemicals. Need more be said?

Unsightly cracks on the fingers and around the nails can be caused by too much exposure to cold, dry air. Gloves aren't only smart fashion accessories; they also protect the skin while keeping the hands warm. Chapped hands aren't only unattractive, they sting like crazy. Applying a hand cream before exiting into the cold and when coming back inside after frigid exposure always makes sense. Obviously, so does protecting them with gloves. Even in mild weather,

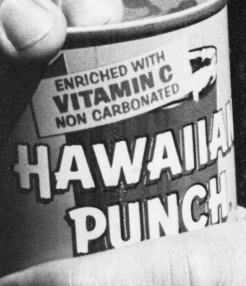

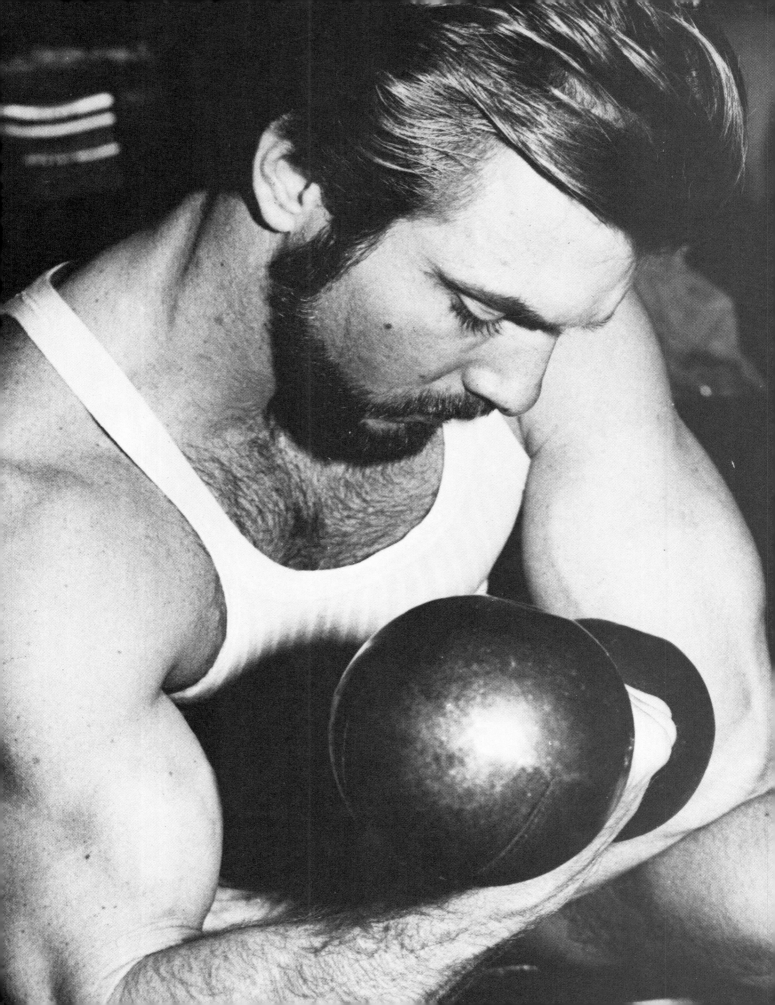

cycling gloves cut down on blister-inducing friction between hands and handlebars while also securing your grasp. Gardening gloves keep the damp soil at a cleaner distance while also sheltering the skin from the sun's rays.

If you're a Klutz and are constantly burning or bruising yourself, cut it out. Go to charm school; learn some poise. You can't go around wearing gloves forever, and how else can you hide those eyesores?

Even though they're seldom underused, hands may require exercise too. Particularly when they are overused and feel cramped. One of the most revitalizing exercises involves simultaneously trying to touch all your fingertips to the points where your finger joints meet the upper pads of your palm, then quickly flexing the fingers out in full extension. Let the fingers dangle for a moment's relaxation, then repeat the routine several times.

CHAPTER 29

WEATHER VAIN
SEASONAL CONSIDERATIONS

Nobody sings the praises of hands and feet. Song lyrics rhapsodize about many splendored eyes, faces, hair, bodies. Hands and feet, never. *Whoops!* There's a song called "Little Hands" from the floppola Broadway musical, *Anya*. And "The Emperor's Thumb" from the forgotten television production of Androcles and the Lion. And from another all-time winner with the same title, there's "Walking Happy." So much for that theory. But feet and hands are hardly in the "Heart and Soul" category. Let's hope that year-round you give them more thought than lyricists do.

THE FRIENDLY SKIES
SPRING & FALL

Maybe most of us don't wax warmly about hands and feet because there's not a helluva lot to do specially for them, other than fitting them into handsome gloves or comfortable shoes, washing and soothing them, exercising them, and keeping their nails neatly clipped.

Nevertheless, a few novelties do exist. Having a professional manicure and pedicure is a nice way to greet the friendly seasons. What else? You could buy a foot massager, since you'll probably be spending more time hiking. Oh! and you can make sure that you don't get them in poison ivy. If you do, wash them with brown laundry soap. Instead of salving them with Calamine lotion, one prominent dermatologist promotes applying the afflicted areas with cool compresses soaked in equal amounts of water and skim milk. Who knows why, but it sounds eccentric.

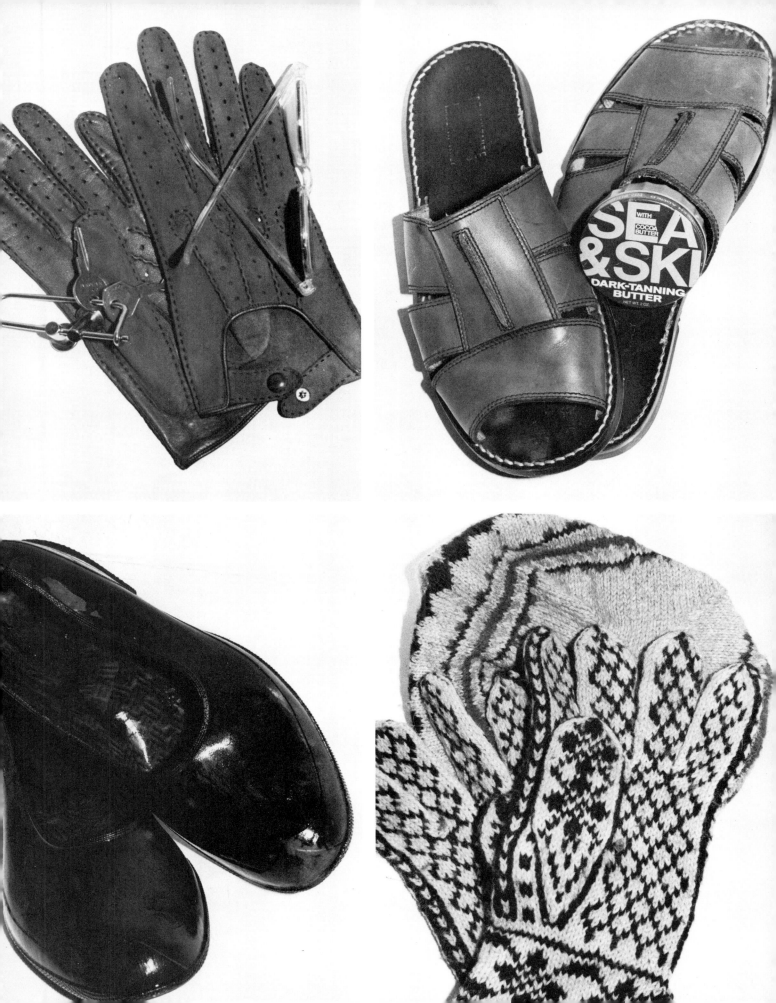

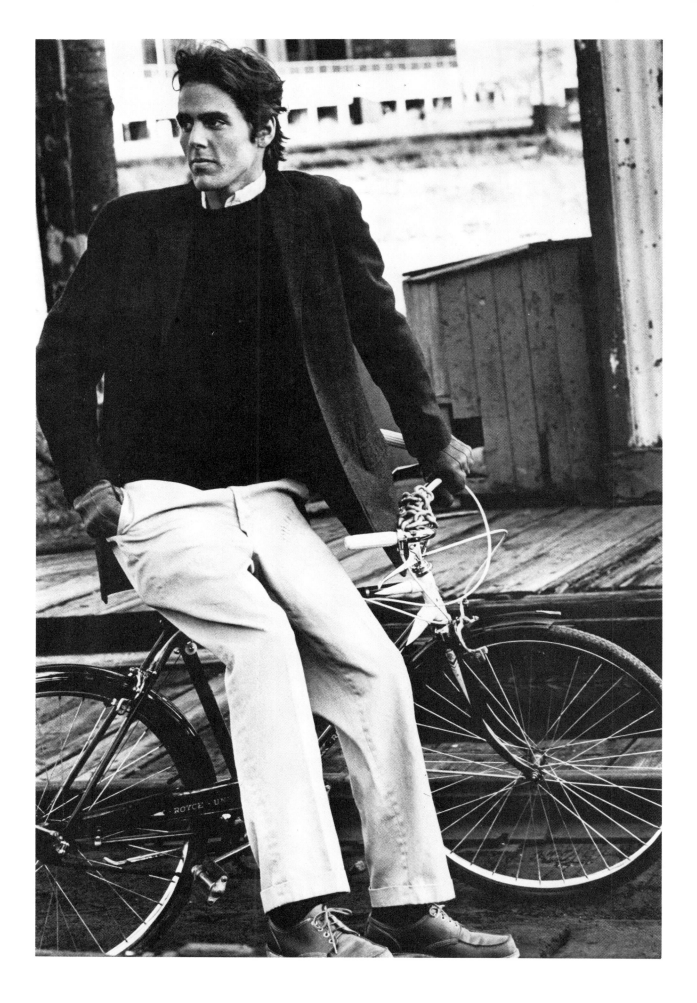

THE COLD WAR
WINTER

Odds are you won't go barefoot in wintry gales, so you probably needn't worry too much about frostbite. On the other hand—or foot—sweaty socks are more worth worrying about. As noted earlier, miliaria is a condition marked by those little blistery bumps that arise when perspiration becomes imprisoned under the skin without escape. On the feet, these little fellows become bigger and even more sweat filled. Skiers who wear several pairs of socks and don't remove them inside the lodge are susceptible. So is the businessman who trots about town without galoshes, gets his feet wet, then goes back to his office. If the wet socks don't dry quickly enough, problems.

Whenever hands are exposed to the cold, they should be treated with a hand cream both before and after each encounter, as previously noted.

Back to your feet. Lightly pumicing them every night helps eliminate the rough spots that seem unavoidable in winter. Remember, soothe them afterward with a lubricant.

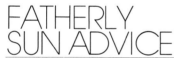

FATHERLY SUN ADVICE
SUMMER

Certain potential problems for hands and feet threaten throughout the year but are more likely to materialize during warm weather.

Since you're actively partaking of the sporting life, you may experience blisters. They occur when something traumatic to the skin happens. The occasion may be as simple as cycling. Somehow the outer and inner skin layers become separated by some physical force, probably friction. Then chemicals are released in the skin; some blood vessels may spring a leak. Since red blood cells are too big to ooze out, only a less voluminous clear liquid (endema fluid or serum) escapes. If the resulting blister isn't too large or painful, leave it alone. As long as it stays closed, it will remain sterile. However, when it takes on sizable dimensions, it's safer to puncture it yourself, since that way you can take precautions to keep it clean. Grandma's method of bursting blisters is still the best: Sterilize a pin over a flame, then zap that ol' blister twice to accommodate drainage. Unfortunately, Grandma used to forget to apply an antibacterial ointment and to cover the deflated blister with a bandage. Don't you make that same mistake.

Weekend athletes often discover that one or several of their toenails have quickly turned alarmingly black. The black plague? No, what's commonly called tennis toe. It's really a blood hemorrhage (less serious than it sounds) under the toenail, probably caused by stubbing the toe or making stops too quickly, thereby jamming the toes into the shoes. The discoloration moves out with growth. Unless your nails are whiz kids, it may take six months or so before the color is totally clipped away. The only way to disguise it is to paint your toenail. Forget it.

The palms, like the soles, are riddled with sweat glands. Sweaty palms are a nuisance, but there's little you can do about them. Hot weather has less to do with the problem than heated-up emotions. Try to get your head together, and overly sweaty palms will stop being a hand-wringing aggravation.

In fact, achieving a relaxed mental and emotional state will eliminate many grooming distresses. However you get there—be it meditation, healthy sex, or being reborn—it doesn't matter. Getting there does. Internal contentment does wonders for the exterior.

APPENDIX

MANUFACTURERS & MAIL ORDER SUPPLIERS OF MEN'S GROOMING PRODUCTS

Many companies either sell men's grooming products by mail order or will answer grooming questions by mail. Considering how many firms are involved in the men's grooming market, a complete listing would be impracticable. Following is a compilation of some firms that are especially responsive to mail inquiry. Being listed does not mean endorsement by either the author or the publisher.

Although mail order companies are specified below, there's absolutely no reason why a man should feel queasy about approaching men's—or even woman's—cosmetic counters to ask for information or demonstrations on how products are to be used. Numerous fine and effective grooming products are packaged and scented for men and in most cases are sold in retail stores. However, women's products may be more readily available. Who gives a shrug if a moisturizer is packaged in pink posies if its fragrance isn't nauseating and if it works? Remember, if you got the guts—and you should have—to approach a women's cosmetics counter and the saleslady laughs, she's the chauvinist sow. Anyway, she won't laugh. Having a neat-looking guy like you at her counter will relieve the monotony and make her day.

Alex Young, Inc.
27 Pleasant Street
Box 1126
Brockton, Massachusetts 02401
617-588-1146

Available only by mail order, their products are used together to form a skin care system that includes conditioning and texturizing. Two small samples are provided free with information about the line. "Quick Change" products is this firm's phrase for "makeup." The informative brochure is well put together and quite specific.

Aloe Creme Laboratories
2104 West Commercial Boulevard
Ft. Lauderdale, Florida 33310
800-327-7673

The maker of tanning products also manufactures assorted skin care items. Products are not sold by mail, but the firm will supply free printed information to those requesting it.

Amora Industries, Inc.
139 East 57th Street
New York, New York 10022
212-752-6140

Hairpieces sold in salons and barber shops. Also available by mail. Will provide printed material about their pieces.

Andromeda, Inc.
P.O. Box 1A
Minnetonka, Minnesota 55343
612-448-4181

Bath products by mail, plus items for body care, fragrances, cosmetics.

Ann Keane Skin Care
16 West 57th Street
New York, New York 10019
212-586-2803

A private salon located only in New York City. Products sold by mail order. The brochure is aimed at women, but clearly defines Ms. Keane's theory of skin care.

Aramis, Inc.
767 Fifth Avenue
New York, New York 10022
212-826-3700

Probably the maker of the world's most extensive men's grooming line, Aramis does not sell its products via the mail. The company will supply free information about generic grooming subjects as well as suggested usage of grooming aids marketed. Aramis makes colognes, aftershaves, soap, muscle soaks, deodorants, antiperspirants, shampoos, conditioners, moisturizers, you name it.

Caswell-Massey Co. Ltd.
518 Lexington Avenue
New York, New York 10017
212-755-2254

The oldest apothecary in America, Caswell-Massey offers its extensive catalogue for $1. It's very kicky. The 1976–1977 one, for example, is "dedicated to famous people who have bathed, bothered and bewildered themselves with the fascination of fragrance, with beauty and well-being." Products for virtually all grooming techniques are included and sold by mail.

Clairol, Inc.
345 Park Avenue
New York, New York 10022
212-644-3020

Clairol makes numerous hair products for men, none of which are sold by direct mail. However, the firm maintains a "Clairol Hot Line" to answer consumer inquiries directly on all matters related to hair. A staff of ten consultants is available Monday through Friday, 9:00 a.m. to 5:00 p.m. (New York time) by calling 800-223-5800 toll free. (New York residents: 212-644-2990.) Readers who prefer to write should address their letter to Clairol Consumer Consultants, 345 Park Avenue, New York, New York. A free male hair care pamphlet, "Your Hair—Make the Most of It," is available upon request by writing to the same address and mentioning the brochure by name. Although aimed primarily at teen-agers, it does include some useful information for adults, plus helpful hints for using blow dryers, which Clairol also manufactures.

Jacqueline Cochran, Inc.
630 Fifth Avenue
New York, New York 10020
212-489-2430

This firm distributes the Pierre Cardin fragrance line, which includes a face-saving aftershave balm. Well-versed in handling written inquiries, the company will also send small (5/8-ounce) samples if requested and if in stock.

Door 26
3131 Southwest Freeway
Houston, Texas 77098
713-526-2686

Foldable pocket moustache scissors.

Dorian Grey
201 Park Avenue
Birmingham, Michigan 48009
313-642-2070

Mail order exclusively. Will provide information on products upon request.

Electrolysis Society of America, Inc.
1540 Broadway
New York, New York 10036
212-757-6300

A hair removal salon.

Fabergé Inc.
1345 Avenue of the Americas
New York, New York 10019
212-581-3500

The company, which makes Brut and Macho fragrance and skin products, does not sell by direct mail. In addition to its retail lines, Fabergé has created a professional line which is sold in hair salons.

Germaine Monteil
40 West 57th Street
New York, New York 10021
212-582-3010

Maker of the Realm men's fragrance line, the company makes a limited number of grooming products for males. No mail order. Free information upon request, including product information on women's products that are applicable.

Hair Again Ltd.
14 East 60th Street
New York, New York 10022
212-832-1234

Specializing in hair implantation, this firm will supply excellent and extensive material about its technique. Question-and-answer sheets include medical, financial, and technical subjects. A comprehensive brochure is also available upon request. Hair products for replacement hair are sold via the mail.

Hair Club for Men Ltd.
185 Madison Avenue
New York, New York 10016
212-889-9290

Specializing in hairweaving, the company also has an excellent and comprehensive brochure available free of cost.

Headstart Hair for Men
240 Madison Avenue
New York, New York 10016
212-686-6040

Specializing in wigs and hairpieces, the firm distributes its goods nationally in hairstyling salons as well as offering them by direct mail. It also offers shampoos and conditioners for replacement hair. It offers a good pamphlet for free.

Imré Gordon Electrolysis, Inc.
8380 Melrose Avenue
Suite 304
Los Angeles, California 90069
213-651-1615

Will provide fact sheets about the process of hair removal, but this is a private electrolysis studio in only this one location.

Klinger for Men
501 Madison Avenue
New York, New York 10022
212-751-9590

Georgette Klinger is probably America's most famous facialist. She operates salons in Beverly Hills and Bar Harbor as well as New York. Her products are available only within her salons and by mail. The free brochure contains more information about men than the others as well as succinctly presenting her case for professional care.

Mario Badescu Skin Care
320 East 52nd Street
New York, New York 10022
212-758-1065

An exclusive salon. Privately formulated products are available by mail after a skin analysis questionnaire is filled out. A handsome brochure is available free, which, although geared primarily to women, does explain the Badescu philosophy well while offering a rundown on his products.

Mary Quant Cosmetics Ltd.
450 Park Avenue
New York, New York 10022
212-644-1234

The famous designer has created a makeup kit for men that is available by direct mail. Send queries to the above address.

MEM Company, Inc.
Union Street Extension
Northvale, New Jersey 07647
201-767-0100

The maker of English Leather cologne as well as other men's fragrances, MEM offers a variety of grooming products—cleansing, shaving, hand and body care—that are scented for compatibility. Free written material is limited to an illustrated catalogue and a price list. Not in the mail order business, MEM will accept a mail order for direct shipment only when the merchandise is not conveniently available in a shopping area.

Mr. Rick Cosmetics for Men
Box H
Melrose, Massachusetts 02176
617-233-2040

Cosmetic products, with the emphasis on eyecolorings, plus cleansing products, which are available in some men's styling salons. Primarily mail order. Information on the products is provided on request.

Meyrowitz Opticians
520 Fifth Avenue
New York, New York 10036
212-682-3880

The retail firm specializing in fashion eyewear has an excellent brochure about choosing appropriate eyewear to complement facial shape. It is available free upon written request.

Nickolaus Exercise Centers
275 Madison Avenue
New York, New York 10016
212-679-7205

A brochure costing $2 explaining the technique is available. Entitled "Exercise For Men," the pamphlet emphasizes breathing, abdominals, and various exercises for strength and flexibility.

Norelco
100 East 42nd Street
New York, New York 10017
212-697-3600

The maker of electric shavers, blow and styling dryers, curling wands, and assorted skin and cleansing implements does not make its products available by mail order, but free printed information will be sent to those requesting it.

Ogilvie
680 Fifth Avenue
New York, New York 10019
212-247-4100

The firm specializes in hair care products. Although the company does not have printed brochures available, attempts will be made to answer written information requests addressed to the Public Relations Department.

The Pantene Company
240 Kingsland Road
Nutley, New Jersey 07110
201-235-4133

Products available nationally in better drug and department stores. If not available locally, the company will sell the products via mail order. Free brochures available, including one on choosing brushes and one entitled "Hair—and How to Care for It."

Perfumer's Workshop Ltd.
1 East 57th Street
New York, New York 10022
212-759-9491

Essential oils and solutions for mix-your-own colognes. Also finished fragrances. Sold in department and specialty shops, the products are also available by mail. Free printed information provided upon request.

Sal Michael Studio
19 East 57th Street
New York, New York 10022
212-421-8043

Hair and scalp products available by mail. Information on products and their use available upon request.

Scannon, Ltd.
666 Fifth Avenue
New York, New York 10019
212-246-3070

Maker of the cologne Kanøn, Scannon also makes a number of grooming products for body, skin, and hair that are distinguished by the Kanøn scent. Products are not sold via mail order, but the company will supply the name and address of local stores that will fill such requests. With the response comes a small sample packet of the fragrance, plus printed product information.

Total Man Laboratories
525 Main Street
Fort Lee, New Jersey 07624
(Will not accept phone orders.)

Although sold in some retail stores, their facial care products (a list is available upon request) are primarily mail order items.

Tuli-Latus Perfumes Ltd.
146-36 13th Avenue
Whitestone, New York 11357
212-746-9337

Fragrance "reproductions," including perfume for men. Sold only via mail order. A free brochure available.

INDEX

A

U

Ultrasonic scalp stimulation, 10
Ultraviolet rays, 82, 127, 172, 175
Unclean underwear, 140
Underweight, being, 155
U.S. Food and Drug Administration, 156

V

Valmy for Men, 206
Vandyke beard, 60
Vitamin A, 156–157
Vitamin B$_1$, 156
Vitamin B$_6$, 156
Vitamin C, 156
Vitamin D, 156–157
Vitamin E, 156
Vitamin Information Service, 206
Vitamins, 155–156, 177
   RDA recommended allowance, 156
Vitiligo, 175

W

Walking briskly (exercise), 164–165
Walrus moustache, 58
Warts, surgical removal of, 123
Water jets (nozzle attachments), 135
Water skiing, 167
Waxing, 150
Weight lifting, 164, 165

Whirlpools, 169
Whiteheads, 82–83
Wigs, 42–45
   advantages of hairpieces over, 48
   difference between toupees and, 42
   procedure for buying, 44–45
   pros and cons of, 45
   shade and color, 44
Windburned lips, 117
Winter, seasonal considerations for:
   body care, 170–172
   hair care, 66
   hands and feet care, 199
   skin care, 126–127
Witch hazel, 92
Wrinkle prevention (factors to consider), 98–103
   aging, 103
   cigarette smoking, 100–102
   cosmetic, 100
   environmental, 98
   exercise, 100
   moisturization, 100
   rest, 102–103
      See also Cosmetic surgery

Y

Yogurt, 157

Z

Zervoulei, John, 42–45
Zinc oxide, 117